T0032356

The Secret World of Stem Cell Therapy

Praise for The Secret World of Stem Cell Therapy

This book by Dr. von Schwarz explains whatever one needs to know about stem cell therapy, easy to understand and scientifically sound.

Frank Stallone, Musician, Los Angeles, USA

Great read for those who want to learn more about stem cells or regenerative medicine.

Fabio, Model, Los Angeles, USA

Refreshing, informative, scientific, and very helpful. Finally, a useful tool helpful from an expert in the field for all of us prospective patients on everything one needs to know on stem cell therapy.

Drea de Matteo, Actress, New York, USA

Dr. Schwarz's book on stem cells is a long-awaited insiders perspective based on years of clinical and research experience. This text will replace hours of internet research as well as initial discussion with less informed medical professionals. Highly recommended.

Prof. Laurent Cleenewerck, Theologian, Washington DC, USA

As a patient of Dr. Schwarz, I found his book highly informative. Additionally, I received stem cell therapy and I experienced what I would consider to be truly miraculous results.

Pete Angelus, Music Producer, Phoenix, USA

A reliable source of the untold truths about a revolutionary topic in medicine by one of the most qualified experts. Thank you for all you do.

Liliana Mattaeus, Model, Munich, Germany

I have known Dr. Ernst Schwarz for many years as an exceptional Cardiologist. His research on Stem Cell Therapy is worth reading for those who are considering its use.

Frank G. Mancuso, Studio Executive, Los Angeles, USA

A great guide to navigate the science, regulations, and pitfalls of one of the most promising medical breakthroughs of our time.

Dr. Parag Bharadwai, Physician, Irvine, USA

The SECRET WORLD of STEM CELL THERAPY

What YOU Need to Know about the Health, Beauty, and Anti-Aging Breakthrough

Prof. Dr. Ernst von Schwarz

NEW YORK

LONDON • NASHVILLE • MELBOURNE • VANCOUVER

The Secret World of Stem Cell Therapy

What YOU Need to Know about the Health, Beauty, and Anti-Aging Breakthrough

© 2022 Prof. Dr. Ernst von Schwarz

All rights reserved. No portion of this book may be reproduced, stored in a retrieval system, or transmitted in any form or by any means—electronic, mechanical, photocopy, recording, scanning, or other—except for brief quotations in critical reviews or articles, without the prior written permission of the publisher.

Published in New York, New York, by Morgan James Publishing. Morgan James is a trademark of Morgan James, LLC. www.MorganJamesPublishing.com

Proudly distributed by Ingram Publisher Services.

Dr. Ernst von Schwarz is President and Owner of "Ernst Schwarz, MD A Professional Medical Corporation," Los Angeles, California, President and Owner of "Pacific Heart Medical Group," Murrieta, California, and Chief Medical Officer of "HeartStem, Inc.," Beverly Hills, California.

Medicine and medical science are in constant flux. The statements made in this book represent the personal opinion of Dr. Ernst von Schwarz but do not replace any recommendations or prescriptions from any healthcare professional to any patient. In addition, the statements do not represent a complete review of the current scientific data on stem cell therapy but an overview to the best of the Dr. Ernst von Schwarz's knowledge at the time of writing.

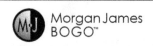

Morgan James BOGO™

A **FREE** ebook edition is available for you or a friend with the purchase of this print book.

CLEARLY SIGN YOUR NAME ABOVE

Instructions to claim your free ebook edition:
1. Visit MorganJamesBOGO.com
2. Sign your name CLEARLY in the space above
3. Complete the form and submit a photo of this entire page
4. You or your friend can download the ebook to your preferred device

ISBN 9781631957079 paperback
ISBN 9781631957086 ebook
Library of Congress Control Number: 2021942516

Cover & Interior Design by:
Christopher Kirk
www.GFSstudio.com

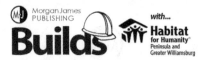

Morgan James is a proud partner of Habitat for Humanity Peninsula and Greater Williamsburg. Partners in building since 2006.

Get involved today! Visit MorganJamesPublishing.com/giving-back

Dedicated to

Aubriana D'Ivana Angel, Lujain Vanessa, Cecilia Florence Magdalena, Nathaniel Ferdinand Valentino, and Rafferty Atticus Kip von Schwarz

Table of Contents

Acknowledgments

This book is a synopsis of more than twenty-two years of work in basic research as well as clinical studies using stem cell therapy for different conditions. Research is always made possible by teamwork, which includes extensive brainstorming, idea development, formulation of study protocols, many hours day and night of study conduction, as well as analysis interpretation and preparation of scientific manuscripts.

I hereby would like to thank my business partner and coworker in our stem cell business, Mrs. Karen Mulholland Angelus for her continued dedication and always positive energy, as well as many of our collaborators, coworkers, researchers, and assistants for their dedicated work both in the past and ongoing. In particular, I would like to thank Dr. Nathalie Busse, Dr. Paul Bogaardt, Jenny Rodstein, Meg Gomez, Maria Gonzalez, and Batuhan Kutlu.

I was inspired by my former professors to dive into the research of stem cell therapies, in particular the outstanding and highly decorated scientist **Prof. Dr. Wolfgang Schaper,** former director of the Max Planck Institute for Experimental Cardiology, Bad Nauheim, Germany, who is one of the most intellectual academics in the world, and his wife,

Prof. Dr. Jutta Schaper, from the same institute, **Prof. Dr. Peter Hanrath**, former director of the Department of Cardiology, RWTH University Hospital Aachen, Germany, who guided me to complete my thesis and become a professor after the habilitation, **Prof. Dr. Robert Kloner**, former director of the Heart Research Institute, Good Samaritan Hospital and the University of Southern California (USC), Los Angeles, California, US and **Prof. Dr. Barry Uretsky** former director of Cardiology at the University of Texas Medical Branch (UTMB), Galveston, Texas, who both showed me the importance of a systematic approach to any scientific problem, and **Prof. Dr. PK Shah**, former Director of Cardiology, Cedars Sinai Medical Center, Los Angeles, who brought me back to Los Angeles and became a clinical scientist role model for me and many others.

I would like to thank Morgan James Publishing for helping me to bring this book to life.

I also would like to thank my late parents, Ernest Johann Ferdinand v. Schwarz and Frieda Elise v. Schwarz, for their support in pushing me to research whatever sounds impossible and my wife, Angela, and my children for their patience and support to get the publication completed.

Preface

Stem cell therapy is considered to be the most important discovery in modern medicine, likely bigger than the discovery of penicillin or the detection of the tuberculous bacteria. It is the path to rethinking the traditional dogmas of several pathophysiologic concepts. It also made us reconsider the definitions and meaning of cell death, processes of aging and degeneration, and the natural course of diseases. Tons of scientific data is published about the benefits of stem cell therapy; however, its widespread practical use is intentionally prohibited by government regulators like the FDA to protect patients from unapproved therapies with a lack of large-scale clinical and scientific data. On the other hand, thousands of businesses currently make big money from desperate patients who believe an internet ad for stem cell therapy as the "cure of diseases" like heart disease and cancer. These ads are often provided by nonscientific individuals and even some healthcare providers.

In order to understand the dilemma of modern stem cell therapy, we must acknowledge the "squaring the circle" challenge. That is the almost-impossible problem of translating reliable basic research into daily clinical practice without accepting business-driven delays introduced by regulatory agencies and the health industry and avoiding companies and providers who sell false promises to patients for thousands of dollars for the cure of diseases without knowing the risks and potential outcomes.

To critically reveal the truth about stem cell therapy apart from overwhelming and false data, we must first evaluate the following five interest groups that are heavily involved in the current practice of stem cell therapy, either directly or indirectly.

Interest Groups for Stem Cell Therapy:

- **Basic Researchers**
- **Clinical Researchers**
- **Healthcare Providers**
- **Stem Cell Companies**
- **Regulatory Agencies**
- **Patients**

Group 1(A): **Basic Researchers**, the "academicians." These are basic researchers who have done tons of work on the pathophysiology of diseases and the efficacy of stem cell injections in experimental (mostly animal) models.

Group 1(B): **Clinical Researchers**, the academic clinicians. These are researchers with a large publication list in their curriculum vitae who know basic research data and some clinical data and are driven by researched funded by the National Institutes of Health (NIH) to establish their working hypotheses. They do not recognize or accept other less-established researchers who might have a lot of clinical experience without the academic reputation.

Group 2: **Healthcare Providers**, doctors, and other advanced care providers. These are providers who use stem cells in their clinical practice for different conditions and who have seen impressive anecdotal successes but have no academic reputation and have never written a scientific paper to publish their observational results. Amongst this group is a subgroup of providers who claim to cure diseases and charge desperate patients a lot of money per injection but never provide follow-up or further testing (the so-called "black sheep").

Group 3: **Stem Cell Companies** and laboratories. These are sometimes created by physicians and researchers without any direct connection to patients and other times created by investors without any ties to medicine, and they sell their stem cell products to physicians for use on their patients. Amongst this group are companies with somewhat shady business ethics and, in several cases, companies that have no doctors or researchers on their teams but consist purely of businesspeople interested in their own financial profit with no regard for patient safety or the cleanliness of their products.

Group 4: **Regulatory Agencies**, governmental agencies such as the Food and Drug Administration (FDA) and other regulators. These are mainly financed by the healthcare industry with no interest in supporting or approving new therapies since no large entity lobbies for more research if there is no industrial benefit. On the other hand, these regulatory agencies protect consumers—all of us—against unproven or questionable therapies.

Group 5: **Patients**, consumers, all of us. We are all patients with current or potential diseases and health problems, looking for alternatives or cures when doctors tell us there is none. Consumers often search the internet for answers and are bombarded by an unprecedented amount of uncontrolled, and oftentimes false and misleading, information. We as patients are in the middle of false information and are unable to interpret scientific data or extrapolate shady findings to different populations. We are the ones who need special guidance.

As a physician and scientist, I am going to show you the points of view from these five interest groups. The fact is that I belong to all of these groups, likely more than anyone else in the business. I am a physician and clinical cardiologist, and I take care of very sick patients every day in my clinics as well as in several hospitals, including large academic centers. I am also a researcher and scientist, and I was among the first in the world to perform basic research stem cell studies by using embryonic heart muscle cells and stem cells in experimental animal models to reduce heart attacks. I was actively involved in NIH-funded stem cell studies in patients with heart diseases. I have published more than 150 scientific articles in international peer-reviewed journals, as well as books and book chapters in medicine. I have been a member of stem cell expert committee groups of academic institutions advising regulatory agencies, but I am also involved in the clinical practice of stem cell therapy for a limited number of patients in the frame of smaller clinical studies.

Based on my experience, I will give you, the reader, insights that many may not want to hear—to unveil the truth, the myths, and the secret world of stem cell therapy.

Introduction

This is the one and only book you need to read if you are interested in stem cell therapy, either for yourself or a loved one as a potential patient, or if you just want to look behind the curtains to see the evidence and the reality of today's stem cell research and its promising clinical implications.

Many books have been written by individuals who want to promote their services and sell stem cell therapies. There is a wide discrepancy between what has been published in the scientific literature and what is advertised in the media about stem cell therapies. No other topic in medicine has gained more interest from both serious researchers and the public than the promising treatments using stem cells for a wide variety of both acute and chronic illnesses.

This book's goal is to provide people current knowledge about the secret world of stem cell therapy from the perspective of a researcher and clinician who has a wide array of experience in the basic research lab, clinical studies, and daily clinical practice treating patients with life-threatening conditions.

Even though I personally use stem cells to treat patients with certain conditions, this book is in no way meant to sell my services. In contrast,

I would like to warn you not to blindly believe in unapproved stem cell therapies presented in an overwhelming amount via internet advertising. Most of these lack any scientific evidence and are presented by people without any scientific or appropriate clinical background.

The book is written based on my personal experiences. I may unintentionally throw some practitioners or companies under the bus, but unless something was public knowledge, I avoided using real names.

For the consumers, the patients, all of us, this book should serve as a guide for how to approach promising new treatments without relying on information provided by a single person or advertiser. It is also meant to help readers develop critical thinking before spending lots of money on questionable therapies. It should also make readers realize that the FDA as a regulatory government entity is not infallible and is often guided by lobbyist interests. Unfortunately, many of us do not have the luxury of being able to wait twenty or more years for a regulatory agency to finally approve a therapy that has the potential to save and preserve thousands of lives.

This book reveals the secrets and sorts the scientific facts of current stem cell research and critically demonstrates the basics of published studies, including some shortcomings. I discuss the reasons why "big pharma" has little interest in stem cell therapy and why insurance companies are not going to pay for it—and likely won't for the next twenty-five years—unless the public and insured customers put pressure on them, which is overdue.

I also explain the current practice of doctors offering indistinguishable stem cell therapies for everyone (It is never true that everything works for everyone, by the way!). I also discuss the myths and truth behind "anti-aging medicine" as a big business and give advice about how to avoid getting caught up in marketing promises. Instead, I try to show readers how to ask the right questions beforehand.

True translational research that leads "from bench to bedside" treatment opportunities is also addressed. These approaches are performed by several scientific groups worldwide in patients using "regenerative therapies" for acute injuries as well as for chronic degenerative diseases. I also describe some of my group's own published and unpublished study data with different outcomes over the last twenty years of research and clinical practice using stem cell therapies.

As a result, I hope readers understand the enormous potential of stem cell therapy in modern medicine. Moreover, I sincerely hope that this book can serve as a guide for those who are interested in stem cell therapies but do not know how to find the right sources and avoid being blinded by nonscientific marketing materials. I try to shed some light on the unknowns, the pitfalls, and the risks, list questions to ask physicians offering therapies, and provide an overview of the current knowledge of stem cell therapy and its huge potential in modern medicine now and in the near future.

Medical science is *in flux*, and there are new developments every day. In no way do I intend to be all-inclusive, neither do I pretend to know everything that has been researched or published on stem cell therapies. My team and I have spent the last twenty-five years participating in basic science and clinical trials using stem cells for different diseases, and we are currently involved in stem cell therapies, scientific analyses of unpublished data, and the preparation of several manuscripts for publication in peer-reviewed scientific journals.

For those who are interested in looking for the scientific reference papers that were used to summarize published data, please see the bibliography.

1.

The Dilemma

- Stem cell therapy might be the biggest breakthrough of our lifetime in modern medicine.
- Large-scale clinical trial data is lacking for broader use of stem cell therapy at this time.

Every single day there are stories published about stem cell therapy. These stories are either in support of it—or harshly against it. There is no middle ground. In fact, there is a current trend that reveals that several groups have no interest in the scientific facts and will not support any form of acceptance by regulators.

Who are these interest groups? Well, they (obviously) include the pharmaceutical industry, parts of the government, the FDA, some insurance companies, some established academic institutions and professional societies, doctors who are not educated about stem cell therapy, some hospitals, nursing homes … the list goes on. Essentially, the groups are comprised of everyone who might benefit from all of us being sick patients, especially if we were suffering from chronic diseases. Why would anyone who profits from sick patients promote a therapy that has the potential to delay the processes of aging and the progression of chronic diseases? That would be counterproductive to their businesses, wouldn't it?

On the other hand, one might argue that it is in everyone's best interest for us to stay younger, healthier, and stronger by natural means using the biologic reserve nature provided—that which is silent and untapped within our bodies. Stem cells are not pharmaceutically engineered; they come from either someone's own body or from pooled donors (placenta or umbilical cord); thus, they have no artificial chemicals in them.

With that being the case, why are we not jumping on it? Why is the FDA shutting stem cell clinics down? Why aren't insurance companies paying for therapies that can save lives and reduce costs down the road? Why are academic institutions staying away from practical applications outside clinical trials? Why are primary practitioners not referring patients to (the few) specialists who have seen the benefits and treat patients with stem cells despite lack of FDA approval?

There are several things that answers all of the above questions. Some make sense. Many include fear of economic downfall. In this chapter, I discuss the pros and cons of stem cell therapy, its current practice, its economic abuse, its enormous potential (based on published data from the scientific literature, my team's research, and clinical data collected over twenty years using stem cells in experimental animal studies, clinical trials, and practical therapies). I will also launch a thorough investigation into the current issues concerning stem cell therapies from a scientific, clinical, regulatory, and qualitative point of view.

Stem cell therapy as a form of modern medicine appears in the news on a daily basis, whether in print, on TV news reports, or on social media. As physicians dealing with very sick patients, especially those with heart and cardiovascular diseases, my colleagues and I are constantly confronted with questions from patients and their caregivers about whether stem cell therapy is an option for them as an additional treatment to the armamentarium of standard therapies.

Simultaneously, we see news reports on stem cells as a "cure" for diseases such as HIV. In the early 2000s, a man named Timothy Ray Brown, first known as the "Berlin patient," was treated with stem cells and remains free of the HIV virus years later. On March 5, 2019, the journal *Nature* reported a second patient who is now free of HIV after stem cell therapy.

But there are also weekly reports of the closure of stem cell clinics by the federal government, especially the FDA. On January 18, 2019, vox.com stated, "the FDA is going after stem cell clinics that peddle unproven treatments." Other news outlets have reported serious side effects, such as the hospital admissions of a dozen patients in three states who received stem cell therapies (mainly intravenously) that resulted in infections from the cell products being contaminated with E. coli and other bacteria (article from *The Washington Post*, December 21, 2018).

These reports are in contrast to the widely publicized anecdotal reports of enormous improvements for different conditions after stem cell treatments. For example, you've most likely seen the video of a dog unable to walk because of chronic hip degeneration and then that same dog was able to happily jump up and down the stairs after stem cell injections.

At the same time, well-known academic institutions also demonstrate and publicize initial results from successful stem cell therapies. On October 11, 2018, physicians and researchers from the University of Southern California Los Angeles (USC) promoted the case of twenty-year-old Kris Bosen from Bakersfield who had a terrible motor vehicle accident that left him permanently paralyzed from the neck down. However, after receiving stem cell injections in his spine as part of an experimental study, Kris regained the use of his hands and arms as evidenced by pictures of him lifting a barbell.

Without a doubt, results like Kris's are life-changing and create hope for thousands of patients with similar conditions who have not been lucky enough to benefit from the potential of experimental procedures, so far.

Stem cell use may be the biggest scientific and medical breakthrough for humankind, but the lack of large-scale randomized controlled study data, the undifferentiated and relatively expensive sale and marketing of stem cell therapies by providers outside of the academic world with no scientific background, and the active attempts by the medical industry and regulatory institutions to avoid the broader use of stem cell therapies for the public has led to confusion, misinterpretation, and pseudo-knowledge for many people trying to understand it.

1.1 The Beginning of Stem Cell Therapy

As a faculty member at major academic institutions with well-established scientific reputations, I have been working on stem cell therapies since 1995. Our group was among the first in the world to use embryonic cells to mimic the effects of stem cells in experimental animal models. For example, we removed embryonic hearts from pregnant rats and injected them in recipient animals that had experimentally induced heart attacks weeks earlier. By injecting male embryonic cells into female recipients, we were able to detect the Y chromosome (male chromosome) as proof that the cells came from the cell injections. Not only did our group show that these cells survived several months after the injections, but we also showed that the extent of the scar tissue from the heart attacks was significantly less, and the contractile function of the hearts injected with cells was significantly better than those treated with placebo injections.[1]

The results of these initial basic research animal studies created hype around the search for the clinical use of stem cells in humans with the design of several clinical trials using different kinds of stem cells for acute and chronic heart diseases as well as other devastating illnesses. Consequently, the first clinical studies using stem cell therapy in patients with heart disease were published in the year 2000 (over twenty years ago).

Precursor cells derived from bone marrow were the first types of cells used in clinical studies in humans with the idea that the transplantation of healthy, multipotent cells would promote the renewal of damaged tissue, the replacement of scars, and the repair of degenerative changes in order to develop into functional cells with an improvement of function (strength) and outcomes.[2]

Despite the fact that every single published study using stem cells has demonstrated benefits—with very little side effects so far—this medical breakthrough has yet to become mainstream for patients in need worldwide. After twenty years and tons of scientific data on the potential and benefits of stem cell therapies, why is this still not an approved therapy?

1.2 How New Therapies Get Approved

To give you an idea of approval processes in the medical community, let me give an example of a drug approval. The drug *nesiritide*, which is meant to treat patients with heart failure, was approved by the FDA in August of 2001 after the evaluation of ten total trials that included 941 patients, including the so-called VMAC trial that looked at 489 subjects with heart failure.[3]

Basically, this drug was FDA-approved for the treatment of acute decompensated heart failure after data showed (only) 489 patients experiencing less shortness of breath compared to standard therapy. It took less than 1,000 patients' data to approve the drug.

Of note, *nesiritide* had fallout years thereafter, and even though it is still approved, it is only used occasionally, in part due to a lack of any long-term benefits and possible negative side effects on the kidneys and the heart.[4]

In other words, a drug that has study data, that is sponsored by a drug manufacturing company, and that reduces shortness of breath for a very short observation period was (relatively) quickly approved by the

FDA for use in humans and subsequently was widely used by physicians—even though no long-term beneficial data was ever seen. So, why was this drug easily FDA-approved and stem cell therapy still awaits approval, despite the fact that thousands of patients have received stem cell therapies all over the world?

Well, let's evaluate the reasons from a scientific and rational point of view. Before doing so, however, please let me assure you that I am not against the FDA or its approval of *nesiritide*. In fact, like many other cardiologists and heart failure specialists, I have been a big fan and frequent user of this drug over the years. My research group even performed an unsponsored clinical trial using *nesiritide* on an outpatient base in patients with chronic heart failure.[5] I am using this drug as a single example to explain the process and the facts of what it takes to get a treatment or drug approved by the FDA.

1.3 Costs of Industrial Support

Stem cell therapy has no industrial lobby because it is not a drug that can be sold by a pharmaceutical company. It will never create trillions of dollars for the industry.

As a natural consequence of business and profitability, the pharmaceutical industry as a whole has to spend money in order to make money. It is not unusual for a pharmaceutical firm to spend several million dollars to conduct a clinical trial. According to a publication from September 2018, the average cost of clinical trials that support FDA approval is nineteen million dollars, which represents only a small portion of the total cost required to develop a new drug.[6] With drug development, preclinical data, animal studies and laboratory studies, and safety and tolerability studies, the average cost for a new drug is estimated at two to three billion dollars. A company only spends that amount of money if the long-term gain exceeds the initial development expenses.

At this point, there is no industrial partner that would benefit from the use of the patients' own stem cells or stem cells derived from donor umbilical cord or placenta tissue. No industry is willing to spend millions or more in clinical studies without the anticipation of financial gains. Therefore, the majority of ongoing stem cell research projects are financed by private, institutional, or federal research funds (such as NIH grants). To receive those "kosher" research grants (how we refer to them in contrast with grants from the pharmaceutical or medical device industry, i.e., those sponsored by an entity that has financial gain in the outcomes of the trial) is not an easy task and usually requires years of research experience and data presentation. Academic researchers, including myself, know very well how difficult it is to get those "kosher" grants after going through the application processes many times over the years.

Not surprisingly, the vast majority of medical breakthrough therapies in this country—and around the world—that are (FDA) approved and recommended per professional society guidelines are, in fact, derived from industrially sponsored clinical trials rather than those sponsored by federal or NIH grants. For example, most of the medical therapies that are part of the standard treatment regimen for the management of patients with a weak heart (heart failure) and are recommended in the guidelines from the American Heart Association/American College of Cardiology and the European Heart Society were based on large-scale clinical trials sponsored by the manufactures of the drugs used in the trials.[7]

Again, I am in no way against the pharmaceutical or medical device industry. In fact, I have performed and participated in several industry-sponsored trials in the past as a principal investigator (more than fifty of them), and I do appreciate what the pharmaceutical industry brings to the advancement of modern medicine. But since I am coming from both worlds—the academic research world and the patient-oriented clinical practice world—I can understand why the industry is not wholeheartedly participating in stem cell research at this time.

1.4 Stem Cell Therapy is Not FDA-Approved

At this point, stem cell therapy marketed and performed outside the bounds of clinical trials in the US **is not** FDA-approved. However, we must distinguish between "stem cell transplantation" and "stem cell therapy." Stem cell *transplantation* has been an FDA-approved procedure for many years in the treatment of certain blood cancers. It does require immunosuppressive therapies to avoid rejection of the transplanted cells, but it can be a highly potent treatment option for certain malignancies.

Stem cell therapy is NOT FDA-approved.

Stem cell therapies by intravenous (IV) injection or tissue injections are quite different from stem cell transplantation. These are usually done without any immunosuppressive therapy, since they are either done from the patient's own stem cells or from donors with a low rejection potential. Many orthopedic doctors and plastic surgeons use injections for joint injuries, arthritis, or facial rejuvenation purposes, among other conditions. This form of stem cell therapy is somewhat FDA "regulated," but it is not FDA-approved.

Again, by no means do I intend to criticize the FDA for not approving uncertain procedures. The FDA is a regulatory agency, and its main task is to protect people from using uncertain and possibly harmful substances or procedures. But we also must keep in mind what determines the approval of a drug or a procedure by the FDA. Leaving out industrial pressure and lobbying, which are hard to prove, it is FDA's job to oversee new therapeutic modalities. Stem cells are not drugs; therefore, I'm not convinced that the FDA in its current model should even be involved in the regulatory processes for stem cells. Instead, since the field of regenerative therapies moves so fast, we should create an independent oversight committee of physicians, regulators, and patient advocates with appropriate experience in these research arenas to regulate and control the broader use of stem cell therapies. If it were left to the FDA, no therapy would be approved unless there was irrefutable evidence of its efficacy, safety, and tolerability with large-scale, randomized, controlled, multicenter trials—as it should be. These trials usually have very stringent inclusion and exclusion criteria in order to ensure a relative homogeneous study population. If healthcare providers who are not used to conducting scientific studies are involved, there are more inconsistencies in patient enrollment and deviations from study protocols in order to enroll more patients. This, of course, contradicts any scientific research process and leads to bias and data invalidity. Even independent of those possible variables, looking at the published data I summarize below, there are so many different patient groups with different diseases and different stem cell therapy protocols using different forms of stem cells via different routes of administration that uniform data is impossible. This, in turn, makes it impossible for the FDA to approve one method of treatment for one condition at this time.

1.5 Lack of Understanding, Lack of Communication

One of the big missing pieces in the stem cell world is a lack of communication and lack of understanding between basic researchers and clinical doctors using stem cell therapies on patients. Those who use stem cells often lack the scientific background for safe use and the ability to create or follow scientific protocols. Further, many (fortunately, not all) providers use stem cell therapies only for monetary gain since this has become a major business for some. In such instances, some providers treat everyone with the same type and number of cells independent of preexisting conditions or possible long-term effects, expecting that the cells perform miracles in a "one-size-fits-all" manner—as long as it is paid for.

Our group, on the other hand, does not believe in this "one-size-fits-all" concept. For example, I don't think a dermatologist should treat a patient with heart failure with stem cell therapy if that dermatologist does not know the basics of heart failure therapy and management. (Unfortunately, I have encountered that exact situation before.)

So, how can a consumer, a prospective patient, or the public in general know where to turn, where to go, and how to get appropriate information about stem cell therapy? I would first say the answer is definitely not from internet search engines or "Dr. Google." But appropriate information is necessary in order to receive clinically indicated therapy that:

1. does not harm,
2. provides the most possible benefits,
3. is not provided by a rip-off,
4. has some existing scientific data on efficacy, and
5. does not interfere with current medicines and treatments prescribed by earlier doctors.

1.6 Words on Anti-Aging

A controversial issue is the often misleading use of stem cell therapy for "anti-aging" purposes. We first need to ask ourselves if there is such a thing as "anti-aging." Aging is a natural process that none of us can escape—at least, not yet. In order to overcome some unwanted "side effects" of aging (such as the loss of elasticity of the skin or the hardening of the blood vessels leading to atherosclerosis (calcification)), a basic understanding of the pathophysiology and morphological and anatomical changes that occur in our bodies' cells during the aging process is essential.

The main side effect of aging is death.
The main risk factor for death is advanced age.

Condemning the concept of "anti-aging medicine" overall is as delusional as the belief in immortality. We do practice concepts of anti-aging, which can lead to a delay of cellular and tissue degeneration rather than an inhibition of aging. But this delay can result in improved quality of life, improve functionality of different organ systems and the organism as a whole, and cause people to look younger and feel better at high numerical ages. The use of stem cell products in the cosmetic industry in creams and gels for skin cell regeneration, for example, lacks scientific proof, and the often-used label "clinically tested" or "clinically proven" has hardly any meaning for a serious researcher unless controlled and reliable study data has been published. But our experience using stem cell therapy for skin rejuvenation over the last twenty years also has shown astonishing results and is currently highly sought by many individuals seeking to look younger and healthier.

Stem cell therapy has been recognized for decades among academicians and has been used for certain blood cancer treatments for approximately thirty years. The concept, however, became more popular in the year 2000 when the so-called clinical landmark studies were published. These studies showed promising repair of damaged organs through regeneration induced by cells that have the ability to develop into special tissues. These cells are the driving factors of human development; thus, they are abundant in embryonic tissue and umbilical cord blood. But some organs in our human body do have the same regenerative powers and can repair damage at least in part, such as the skin and the liver. So, our bodies do contain stem cells for regenerative purposes. We age in part because we lose those regenerative powers, which leads to a loss of the elasticity of our blood vessels, which then results in lack of oxygen, subsequently leading to cellular death—the complete reversal of our organ development in utero and after birth.

So, if the skin and the liver have the ability to regenerate dead tissue, why do other organs in our body not have the same ability? And shouldn't we try to induce such repair mechanisms? That is one of the goals of modern stem cell therapy. It aims to repair damaged tissue by introducing multipotent cells into host organs and having those cells not only survive but actually develop into functional host tissue.

Of note, every single study using stem cells published so far in the scientific literature has shown the benefits of stem cell therapy, but stem cell therapy is still not in widespread use to treat patients. The pharmaceutical industry has no interest in supporting stem cell research; therefore, large-scale studies are lacking. Even many of the academic basic researchers have secondary interests since some own stem cell companies and are interested in their own financial gains. The academic institutions depend on larger translational studies and the disconnect between clinical doctors and laboratory scientists often prevents bench-to-bedside trials from being sufficiently conducted.

The FDA is helpless when it comes to approving therapies without the intellectual property registration processes and regulation procedures typically used by drug companies for new therapies. Many nonacademic or pseudoacademic physicians and their business partners offer unapproved but somewhat regulated stem cell therapies both outside and within the US for cash prizes that cost patients several thousands of dollars. Some of them do not have any research background or pathophysiologic knowledge of cellular processes and lack a clinical reputation amongst their peers for obvious reasons, but they are frequented by celebrities and multimillionaires who believe they can pay enough to live longer. These physicians give the validity of stem cell therapy a bad reputation since they often claim success rates without the experience or capacity to publish their data in a scientific and reproducible manner.

There are others, however, who do have the appropriate scientific background, the clinical expertise and knowledge, and the drive to use available research data for the benefit of their patients with "off-label" therapies. My group sees ourselves among those physicians, and our patients are the ones who usually do not fit into the randomized clinical trials at the academic centers because they are too old and too sick and would skew any trial results. For patients, it is basically impossible to know the difference, since no quality measures or controls exist and, oftentimes, patients are guided by advertising and marketing rather than by professional, scientific, and clinical reputation.

How could anyone know the difference?
As a simple reminder, among other distinguishing features, the good ones usually do not advertise their services on billboards or in magazines.

2.

The Secrets

- Stem cells are power engines, a resource for life, growth, and repair in the living creature.
- Stem cells are undifferentiated cells with the ability to generate, sustain, and replace terminally differentiated cells via unlimited replication.

The human body is made of approximately thirty to fifty trillion cells. Out of those, approximately 300 million cells die every single minute, although cells from different organs have differing life spans. According to a report in *BBC Science Focus*, some of our cells are only replaced every seven to ten years. White blood cells, for example, live for a few days, while skin cells live for a few weeks, liver and pancreas cells live for approximately one year, intestinal (gut) cells live for up to fifteen years (except the cells lining the mucosal surface), heart cells live for several decades (over forty years), cells in the lens of the eyes might last a lifespan, and brain cells might last even longer than the human life (potentially up to 200 years).[8]

There are hundreds of different types of cells in the human body, each with a specific role. For instance, red blood cells carry oxygen, neuron (nerve) cells transmit information to other cells, and skin cells create a protective barrier. In contrast to organ-specific and differentiated cells, stem cells are undifferentiated and capable of 1) replicating themselves, and 2) growing into organ-specific cells. There are two main types of stem cells. Tissue stem cells are found in organs but can usually only create cells of that particular organ. Pluripotent stem cells, on the other hand, can become almost any type of cell in the body.

To understand the uniqueness of stem cells, we must go back to the very beginning of the development of human life: fertilization.

Three days after fertilization, the fetus is simply a clump of thirty-two embryonic stem cells. As the fetus develops, these building blocks of cells multiply and transform into the hundreds of specialized cells found throughout the body: bones, blood, the lungs, the heart, the brain, and so on. Stem cells continue to live in the body—skin, muscles, fat, intestines, and bone marrow—once we are born and they are there until the day we die.

These stem cells are able to reproduce endlessly and are integral in allowing our bodies to grow and heal. However, these adult stem cells are "tissue specific," which means blood stem cells found in bone marrow can only become blood cells (although technically they can become either the white blood cells of the immune system or the red blood cells that carry oxygen).

Stem cells are engines. They are the resource for life, growth, and repair in a living creature. In scientific terms, stem cells are undifferentiated cells that possess the ability to generate, sustain, and replace terminally differentiated cells via unlimited replication. They have two basic features: perpetual self-renewal and capability of differentiation into various phenotypes, depending on the stimuli or signals they receive. Stem cells are commonly subdivided into two main entities: embryonic stem cells and adult or somatic stem cells. A third category of "embryonic-like" cells, also called induced pluripotent cells, are genetically reprogrammed (by pluripotent transcription factors) and have been added in recent years.

Pluripotent stem cells have the capacity to differentiate into all cell types of an organism, including mesodermal derived cardiomyocytes (heart muscle cells). However, in cardiac regenerative medicine, the therapeutic use of pluripotent stem cells is limited because there is risk of immune rejection, genetic instability, potential for forming tumors, low induction efficiency, and ethical issues.

Adult stem cells can further be subdivided into two categories: multipotent (differentiation into unlimited cell types) and unipotent (differentiation into one cell type). Stem cells are named and distinguished by their origin and differentiation capacity. For example, bone marrow derived stem cells (multipotent, including hematopoietic, mesenchymal, and endothelial stem cells) or adipose tissue derived stem cells, among others.

Stem cells are considered to be the initiators and mediators of the repair mechanism in our bodies.

Understanding their adaptive mechanism is essential for conceptualizing how stem cells function. Stem cells have the ability to be pluripotent; that is, they are able to develop into any type of tissue depending on the environmental requirements.

Stem cells also have the potential ability to reverse the death of cells in the human body, a phenomenon that has never been achieved by another form of therapy, to date. The physiologic dogma that cells die and are gone forever means there can be irreversible damage to tissue, usually leading to replacement fibrosis with scar tissue that does not have a function. Organs such as the brain and the heart are especially considered irreplaceable. Any damage caused by strokes or heart attacks can lead to death or permanent disability—without any regenerative power. Current drug treatments focus on prevention by reducing risk factors but deny the existence of natural aging. Getting older is the main reason chronic and degenerative diseases develop—whether that disease is dia-

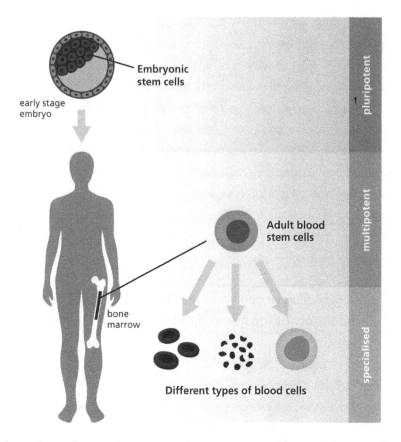

early stage embryo

Embryonic stem cells

Adult blood stem cells

bone marrow

Different types of blood cells

pluripotent

multipotent

specialised

betes, heart disease, dementia, or degenerative conditions of the muscular and skeletal system, just to name a few of the most common ones. None of these conditions can be cured as of today. Once we encounter the condition, we usually deal with the symptoms as best we can until death provides relief.

Besides being the fundamental building blocks of organs, stem cells have the ability to regenerate damaged tissue. For instance, in utero, humans have the ability to fully repair entire organs, such as an extremity (appendage), for up to two weeks after birth. If the tip of a finger is lost or damaged within the first six months of life, we can fully regenerate the entire missing and/or damaged portion of the appendage.

Stem cell

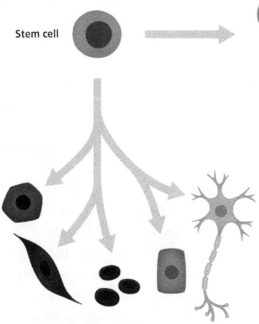

more stem cells

specialised cells

This regenerative property is most likely the reason why, even as adults, we still possess stem cells in our organs, although they have a somewhat limited capacity for self-renewal and regeneration. It appears the evolutionary steps to induce stem cells to perform reparations in case of organ damage are not well-developed yet.

However, we have demonstrated the ability to direct a stem cell's development into the cells of specific organs. For instance, if pluripotent stem cells are deliberately placed in an environment, they respond to benefit the environmental needs as long as the necessary requirements are met. In other words, stem cells have the unique and sophisticated power to achieve the highest levels of adaptability within any living environment.

If stem cells are placed in a suspension of brain cells in a Petri dish in the laboratory, those stem cells develop into neurons (nerve cells); if they are placed in a culture of heart cells, they possess the biological means to develop into active, contractile heart muscle cells (cardiomyocytes); and if they are placed in a suspension of skin cells, they develop into skin tissue (dermatocytes).

As you can see from these examples, stem cells can successfully adapt to any specific organ cells if requirements are provided in a biologically active and viable environment. Similarly, given their capability to repair damage, stem cells provide an opportunity for our bodies to repair biological injuries irrespective of physical location. There are numerous examples of stem cells being used to help heal damaged tissues.

In my team's own experience, we have seen several patients with open wounds on their legs (often secondary to diabetic foot ulcers) that are therapy-resistant to conservative standard treatments. The addition of stem cells applied locally into the tissue or injected in the surrounding tissue resulted in complete healing of the ulcers in many cases.[9]

There are many other examples of improvement to tissue damage with stem cell injections. For example, age-related macular degeneration in the eyes is the most common cause of blindness in adults. The disease erodes the cells responsible for vision in the back of the eye and, until now, no cure was found. In March of 2018, however, two patients regained their vision after receiving a stem cell patch. That patch was created by taking stem cells from an embryo, which had been donated to research, and converting them into retinal cells in a laboratory setting. The stem cells were placed in a special liquid in which they multiplied and, through a process called spontaneous differentiation, turned into various different cell types, including retinal cells. These were then placed on a tiny membrane and injected beneath the patients' retinas.

After a year, both patients—an eighty-six-year-old man and a woman in her sixties—went from not being able to read at all to reading sixty to eighty words a minute with reading glasses. This was achieved by researchers at Moorfields Eye Hospital and the University College London in the UK.

Other researchers have repeatedly proposed that we extract and store our own stem cells at an early age, i.e., while we are young and healthy and possess an abundance of potent stem cells. The idea is that by extracting stem cells from the body, these cells can be used as replacement cells when our parts become damaged or diseased in the future.

These extracted cells can be grown and modified in a laboratory and then transplanted, usually via an injection, back into the body so they integrate with tissue and can aid repair and regeneration. Either the patients' own stem cells are extracted, multiplied in a lab, and reintroduced into the body, or the stem cells come from a donor—either a relative or a stranger.

There are several potential uses for stem cells that are currently being investigated, including breakthrough treatments for debilitating conditions such as multiple sclerosis (a neurological degenerative disease) and Crohn's disease (a disease of the immune system that leads to recurrent bleeding from the intestines). These conditions are driven by the immune system turning against the body and attacking healthy tissue. In these cases, stem cells are used to replace the patients' faulty immune cells with new ones with the hope that the system "reboot" will effectively improve the course of the illnesses.

More recent advances revealed that adult stem cells will also be able to be reprogrammed in a laboratory setting to behave similarly to embryonic stem cells, which would enable them to develop into any cell type in the body. These are known as "induced pluripotent stem cells."[10] Even more exciting, there is mounting evidence that any cell can be modified to become an induced pluripotent stem cell.

That could mean one day a few skin cells could be extracted and used to help build a new heart, lungs, or other body part to be used in a transplant operation. However, we are not there yet.

What about damage to the nervous system instead of various organs?

Superman actor Christopher Reeve was just forty-three years old when he was paralyzed in a horseback riding accident. He was campaigning for stem cell research but died nine years later from complications of the accident. Now, novel stem cell therapies are showing significant benefits in several patients with paralysis.

A team based at the University College London led by Professor Ying Li is actively preparing a clinical trial based on prior work that has already shown improvement of the function of extremities in paralyzed patients. For example, Polish fireman Darek Fidyka recovered his ability to walk despite suffering from a severe injury to his spinal cord.

Work is also ongoing in the US, where nearly thirty patients paralyzed in accidents have been injected with embryonic stem cells in a bid to regenerate their spinal cords. There is cautious optimism with this work. In one group of six patients, four patients gained significant function on one side of their body.

Many other ways of using stem cells to treat different diseases are undergoing clinical trials on patients with encouraging results. Some are even being approved to be given on the British National Health System (NHS).

Given that this is such a new area of medicine, there are obvious concerns about the risks. Therapies that have gone through proper clinical trials are safe for patients, but those not subjected to rigorous tests may not be. Some types of stem cells, such as induced pluripotent stem cells, have great potential but concerns still persist. They appear to be prone to mutating. In some cases, they turn into tumors known as teratomas, and while some mutations may be harmless, others may not be. Further tests are needed to fully understand how stem cells, in particular induced pluripotent stem cells, can be used safely. Stem cells are just like new drugs; they must be rigorously tested before they can be safely used in patients.

Keep in mind that just because one patient experienced improvements in their condition does not mean that the same treatment will work identically on another person. There is no indication or proof of that being the case. As Lord Winston says, "These are very complex areas, and again and again one has to say this technology is still very young indeed. But today, what we can truly say is there is much promise."

There are thousands of examples demonstrating the magnitude of the regenerative powers possessed by stem cells, which are now undoubtedly recognized and accepted by the academic world. However, up to the time of writing this book, there is mainly anecdotal data and only sparse data from small, randomized clinical trials available. Large-scale, placebo-controlled, randomized clinical trials are missing. There is a discrepancy between the promising results of a few patients and the lack of scientific evidence with larger numbers of patients that leaves many aspects of stem cells still a secret.

3

A Simplified Concept

Stem cells are:

- Attracted by damage
- Differentiated into tissue environment
- Damage repair and replacement

In order to explain how stem cells work, let's look at a nonbiological concept. To simplify the idea, we must first assume the following roles of stem cells in order to potentiate their regenerative power:

1. Get into injured or damaged tissue.
2. Work their way to repair.
3. Restore and maintain tissue integrity and function.

In other words, the cells need to get into the environment to be exposed to damaged tissue. Then they use the tissue environment to properly propagate the cells' unique signal mechanisms and develop into functional organ cells, thus their ability to repair and regenerate. In a real-life scenario, however, we have to add another step and change the order from *get in, work, restore* to:

1. Work to get ready.
2. Get into injured or damaged tissue.
3. Work to repair.
4. Restore and maintain tissue integrity and function.

That extra step must be added because to "get in" is work in itself. Given our current generation's evolutionary incompetence, "getting in" is simply not an automated or intuitive biological process. In a biological system, injury is the catalyst for certain cell types to try to repair damage, including cells that improve perfusion (which causes swelling), an inflammatory response, and stem cells to induce repairs. This mechanism, however, is rudimentary at best in most of our organs.

To explain this concept further, imagine your objective is to become a successful lawyer. In order to reach your goal, it is of vital importance that you develop in an appropriate environment conducive to acquiring and developing the necessary skill set and have experiences operating in situations similar to those you will come across in the professional role. For instance, gaining exposure to the accepted behaviors and communication styles necessary to succeed as a lawyer. The initial step and most challenging part of this process is getting admitted into a particular law school that provides adequate resources and learning experiences that support your given professional objectives. Once accepted into a prestigious institution such as Harvard Law School, the process requires additional work—studying, learning, understanding, and professional development—to transform into an effective attorney.

The combination of the appropriate environment and adaptability plus innate capabilities organically develops an individual into a professional with the aptitude to perform the trade effectively. Part of this adaptability is the ability to fulfill academic requirements while operating effectively as a member of the student body, i.e., within the context of rules, regulations, culture, and expectations of the professional culture. Part of this evolution requires an individual to develop in response to the input and feedback from appropriate and specific academic and professional environments, interactions with peers, and observation of those who are already operating successfully in the desired professional role. Over time, this transformative process nurtures an individual's raw intelligence, ambition, and energy and deliberately creates the types of challenges that develop the necessary traits for responding effectively to meet said challenges, thereby allowing time to naturally produce the strengths that create an effective professional.

But, before all of that, the student has to get into law school.

Similarly, the stem cells have to get into the areas of damage first.

Even though there is a natural mechanism by which the damaged tissue signals the body to recruit stem cells for repair, that mechanism is underdeveloped. If it were not underdeveloped, we would not have any chronic diseases since our repair cells would do the job. But obviously, that is not the case. The missing piece is learning how to stimulate the stem cells appropriately and guide them into the areas of interest (like guiding a student to work hard enough to be accepted to a prestigious law school). For these reasons along with the lack of understanding about the exact inductors for cell repair, we are currently showing stem cells where the damage is by injecting them directly into the at-risk tissues, such as using stem cell injections for a patient's knee suffering from arthritis.

Once introduced to the at-risk area, stem cells start exerting their anti-inflammatory capabilities, which results in less pain and improvement of symptoms usually relatively quickly (often within a few days). Furthermore, the stem cells induce angiogenesis, which is the induction of new blood vessel cells leading to the development of capillaries and arterioles (small blood vessels that improve the perfusion and oxygen supply to the tissue).

After that, the cells start differentiating into the recipient's tissue cells to repair damage or replace scar tissue. Keep in mind that this is just the current hypothetical concept of how stem cell injections improve acutely injured or chronically damaged tissues with the lack of better alternatives.

There is consensus that stem cells work by exerting the following properties:

1. Anti-inflammation.
2. Angiogenesis.
3. Regeneration (either directly or indirectly via paracrine effects).
4. Induction of endogenous stem cell activation.[11]

We are still in the early days of understanding how stem cells work, but this concept is the basis for symptom improvements in patients who received stem cell therapies for different conditions.

The Many Unanswered Questions

- Stem cells are not a cure for any disease, so far.
- Stem cells improve symptoms.
- Stem cells possibly delay the progression of chronic diseases.
- We do not know which type of stem cells should be used, nor how often.

I n this chapter, I further explain the types of stem cells that exist. First, for the clinical use of stem cells, it is important to know the difference between *autologous* and *allogenic* stem cells.

4.1 Autologous versus Allogenic Stem Cells

Autologous stem cells are cells provided by patients themselves, meaning that the cells are withdrawn from the patients' own bodies (and then reinjected into the same patients). In this procedure, stem cells can be collected from different tissues, such as bone marrow or fat tissue, and then these cells are injected back into the patient without any major manipulation of the cells. This procedure is called "autologous stem cell therapy." After the cell procurement process, the collected fluid is spun to isolate cells and then the cell suspension is reinjected into the patient. There is no immune reaction anticipated if someone is injected with his or her own cells. This is often used during plastic surgery on the face.

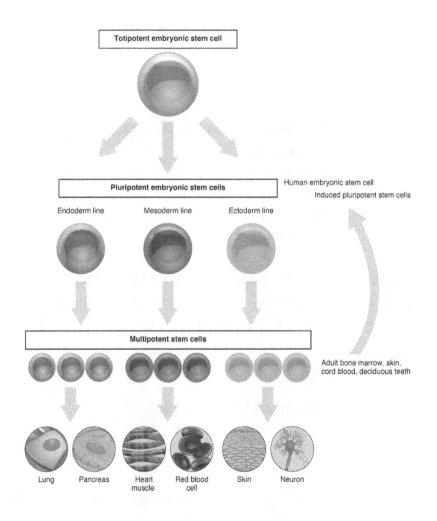

The patients' blood derived stem cells are injected into the skin during or after facial rejuvenation surgeries in order to improve the healing process.

Allogeneic stem cells, on the other hand, are cells from a donor. The theoretical advantage of using donor cells rather than the patient's own cells is that the donor cells usually have much higher potency. For example, using umbilical cord derived donor stem cells, which have everything needed to build entire organs, are much more potent than using a seventy-year-old patient's own (blood derived) stem cells. Stem cells age and lose their regenerative power over time, and both their quality and quantity diminish over time in our bodies' tissues. Therefore, the use of allogenic stem cells has theoretically much more regenerative power than using the patients' own cells. However, allogenic (foreign) cells can theoretically induce an immune response in the recipient after injection.

4.2 Immune Reaction and Antibody Induction

In order to avoid a rejection after receiving an allogenic stem cell injection, the donor's and recipient's human leukocyte antigens should be compatible. However, cells derived from umbilical cord blood or placenta tissue usually do not have any significant antigenicity, meaning that they do not create any clinically significant rejection in the recipient after injection. In other words, there is no relevant immune reaction expected after someone gets allogenic stem cells injected. Even if there was some degree of an immune response, it is usually subclinical, meaning no symptoms are expected. However, any immune response as a result of an IV injection of any blood-derived product could hypothetically lead to the development of antibodies in the recipient. These antibodies would not do any immediate harm, but if the recipient is exposed to another product (such as a transplanted organ in the future), the prior antibody production could create a problem. The same situation exists if a transplant candidate is exposed to a blood transfusion beforehand. As a transplant cardiologist, I deal with organ rejection on a daily base, and in order to avoid the development of antibodies after any blood-product injection (such as stem cells), we actually do not use whole cells for our stem cell clinical studies but acellular allogenic products instead.

Nowadays, many groups, including ours, follow the same process and do not use entire cells. They instead use cellular products such as exosomes (cellular components without cell membranes) that do not induce antibodies in the receiving patients. The catch is that not many studies have been performed to prove that concept. In any case, clinically, it does not cause any problems in the patients immediately as far as we know today. If a patient might need an organ transplant in the future, such as a kidney or a heart, cells injected earlier could induce some antibodies similar to any transfused blood product, which could then make it more difficult to find a matching donor organ for transplantation since the cells could induce so-called human leucocyte antibodies (HLA) that can play a role in transplant organ rejection. By using products without cells—or without cell membranes— this issue becomes nonexistent based on our current knowledge.

4.3 Facts and Questions

Despite all we do know, there are several unanswered questions regarding stem cells in general and stem cell therapy in particular. For example, when used for therapeutic purposes, there is no consensus on which type of stem cell is the best option for which disease, or how many cells are needed and where and how often they should be administered. In contrast to the general opinion that stem cells are a huge mystery overall, below are the current thoughts that are mostly confirmed by scientific leaders in the field of stem cell therapy.

- Stem cell therapy does not cure any diseases but—if used appropriately—might delay the progression of many devastating chronic illnesses.
- Stem cell therapy usually does improve symptoms, pain, and quality of life.
- Stem cell therapy needs to be individualized as well as disease- and symptom-oriented.
- Long-term benefits are possible.
- There are proven benefits for several illnesses.
- Stem cell therapy represents the future of modern medicine and might be the basis for many adjunct treatment options, such as growth factors and gene therapy.

Again, stem cells have not been shown to cure any disease at this point in time (with the exception of stem cell transplantation as a treatment for certain forms of blood cancer). Any claims from healthcare providers that say otherwise are misleading and false.

While we don't know what the best source for stem cells is, there are several sources currently used by different providers to treat disease. I go through the most commonly used stem cell types and sources in the remainder of this chapter.

4.4 Platelet-Rich Plasma (PRP)

Platelet-rich plasma (often referred to as PRP) is derived from the patient's own blood. It is spun down from the patient's blood after thirty to sixty milliliters of blood is taken from an arm vein. There are a few isolation steps, including centrifugation, to concentrate the plasma that contains a lot of platelets.

PRP is a substance that is supposed to promote healing when injected. Plasma is a component of our blood that contains special "factors," or proteins, that help our blood clot. It also contains proteins that support cell growth. The idea is that injecting PRP into damaged tissues will stimulate your body to grow new, healthy cells and promote healing. Because the tissue growth factors are more concentrated in the prepared growth injections, researchers think the body's tissues may heal faster.

Technically, PRP is not the same as stem cells and, per definition, is not a stem cell product. PRP does not contain mesenchymal stem cells or other types of stem cells, but PRP has been shown to speed up repair in injuries (such as joint or muscle injuries) and has been shown to exert anti-inflammatory effects. PRP therapy uses injections of a concentration of a patient's own platelets to accelerate the healing of injured tendons, ligaments, muscles, and joints. In this way, PRP injections use each individual patient's own healing system to improve musculoskeletal problems.

PRP injections are prepared by taking anywhere from one to a few tubes of your own blood and running it through a centrifuge to concentrate the platelets. The average percentage of platelets found in blood is around 6 percent, and the PRP concentration is about 90 percent higher. These activated platelets are then injected directly into injured or diseased body tissue. This releases growth factors that stimulate and increase the number of reparative cells the body produces.

Famous athletes like Tiger Woods and tennis star Rafael Nadal have been known to have PRP injections to help heal injuries, as noted in public statements to the media. PRP may help decrease joint inflammation by modulating synovial cell proliferation and differentiation and inhibition of certain pathways in various skeletal-muscle-joint conditions. PRP has shown good efficacy in osteoarthritis (a chronic inflammation of the bone tissue in several joints, such as the knees, shoulders, and hips) and other musculoskeletal inflammatory conditions such as synovitis and epicondylitis and acute muscle injuries such as strains, sprains, or tendinopathies (tennis elbow).

A recently published review in January 2020 also showed benefits of PRP in patients with chronic degenerative and rheumatoid arthritis during post-surgical recovery. Other data showed some benefits in treating male hair loss with PRP injections (androgenic alopecia).

According to the American Academy of Orthopaedic Surgeons, very few insurance plans will provide any reimbursement for PRP injections. The costs must largely be paid out-of-pocket and can vary from location to location depending on how the injections are used. Some of the reported costs nationwide include:

- *ABC News 7* in San Francisco reports PRP treatments for hair loss cost $900 for one treatment and $2,500 for a set of three treatments.
- *The Washington Post* reports that knee injections of PRP can cost anywhere from $500 to $1,200 per treatment.

Insurance companies consider PRP injections an experimental treatment, which is why it is not typically covered. More scientific research will have to conclude its effectiveness before it is more widely covered. Common side effects or risks of PRP injections include:

- Local or generalized infections.
- Nerve injuries.
- Pain at the injection sites.
- Local tissue damage.

PRP injections are intended to promote healing or growth, and while most patients do not note any difference in their symptoms right away, the injection may promote healing processes within a few weeks.

The treatment has not been definitively proven, and it also has not been approved as a treatment by the FDA.

In our experience, PRP definitely has pro-healing and anti-inflammatory effects, does create a stinging pain when injected, and is an autologous alternative with efficacy but a shorter duration compared to other stem cell therapies.

4.5 Bone Marrow Derived Stem Cells

Everyone involved in stem cell research started by using bone marrow derived stem cells. Bone marrow is the spongy tissue inside the larger bones of the human body that produces red blood cells, white blood cells, and platelets.

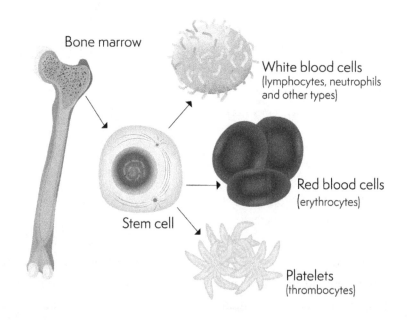

Bone marrow

White blood cells
(lymphocytes, neutrophils and other types)

Red blood cells
(erythrocytes)

Stem cell

Platelets
(thrombocytes)

Using a needle, the aspiration draws out a sample of the liquid portion and a more solid part of the bone marrow. In practical terms, a bone marrow biopsy is performed on the hip bone of the pelvis or the breastbone (sternum) using an invasive approach. After injecting local anesthetics, an aspiration needle is used to go deep in the bone and aspirate the marrow, which takes just a few minutes and might cause some pain. The bone marrow aspirate is then prepared, and bone marrow derived stem cells are isolated in a few separating steps.

Bone marrow derived stem cells, in fact, do represent a heterogeneous group of cells that includes several cell types, including but not limited to, hematopoietic stem cells, mesenchymal stromal/stem cell precursors, and endothelial progenitor cells. Bone marrow derived stem cells are autologous if reinjected into the same patient.

Interestingly, rising amounts of data indicate that bone marrow derived precursor cells may have the ability to differentiate into skeletal muscle cells, heart muscle cells, and cells lining the walls of blood vessels (endothelial cells). The endothelial cells are able to induce the bone marrow to produce blood vessel cells; thus, creating new blood vessels (which is called angiogenesis). These cells are also mobilized into the peripheral blood, giving rise to more mature endothelial cells in newly formed vessels after either injury occurs (such as a heart attack) or within tumors. It has been suggested that the bone marrow serves as a reservoir for the entire body's angiogenesis (along with vasculogenesis, which is the development of larger blood vessels in the body).

As a cardiologist, I am personally interested in these mechanisms since we always attempt to supply jeopardized tissues with blood and oxygen (reoxygenation by means of revascularization through newly developed blood vessels) in cases of strokes or heart attacks. This can improve the function of the brain or the heart after a lack of oxygen from the blockage of a blood vessel causes damage.

There is some indication that human blood vessel precursor cells (endothelial progenitor cells) might circulate throughout our blood system constantly in order to promote new blood vessel development (neovascularization) at sites with lack of oxygen (ischemia, hypoxia, injury, or tumor formation). That means that these cells, in fact, do have the ability to produce vascular tubes and contribute to the functional surface of blood vessels—the endothelial lining of injured or newly developed vascular structures in the living being.

Apart from myocardial and vascular regeneration, other mechanisms of stem cell action have been proposed. In many cases, the frequency of stem cell engraftment and the number of newly generated heart muscle and vascular cells, either through what is called transdifferentiation (the change of appearance and function) or cellular fusion (the conglomeration of cells to from a tissue structure), appear too low to explain the significant functional improvement described in the heart, for example. Accordingly, an alternative hypothesis has been proposed: stem cells release factors that contribute to cardiac repair and regeneration. Indeed, cytokines and growth factors can induce cellular protection and neovascularization. It has also been postulated that paracrine factors may mediate endogenous regeneration via activation of resident cardiac stem cells. Furthermore, cardiac remodeling, contractility, and metabolism may also be influenced in a paracrine fashion.

Let me note that these concepts go way beyond a layperson's understanding of pathophysiological or reparative mechanisms and can even leave scientists baffled. Even now, there is still controversy about whether or not stem cells really do regenerate damaged tissue or whether functional improvements come from the stabilization of healthy (surrounding) tissue caused by some paracrine (indirect supportive) effects.

In experimental animal models, it has been reported that blood cell derived stem cells contributed to the regeneration of heart muscle after direct injection of the cells into the site of an experimentally induced heart attack. Several of these models have documented that transplantation of bone marrow derived stem cell injections after heart attacks is associated with reduction of scar size and an improvement in heart contractile function. There is now clear evidence that bone marrow derived stem cells engraft, survive, and grow within the damaged heart muscle tissue by forming connections with the recipient's heart muscle cells (as measured by the production of connection proteins).[12] Several experimental studies have also shown benefits for inflammatory conditions, spinal cord injuries, heart diseases, and many other illnesses.

Starting with these promising findings, several clinical trials have been conducted analyzing the effects of bone marrow derived stem cell injection in patients with heart attacks who were successfully treated by balloon angioplasty. Likewise, in other trials, patients were treated by direct heart tissue injection during coronary artery bypass graft surgery, mostly in the border zone of formerly damaged heart tissue.[13]

According to a Google search from 2017, the costs for bone marrow derived stem cell injections vary between providers, and I have heard of patients being charged between $2,500 and $7,500 per injection. And according to a poll questionnaire, one-sixth of patients paid more than that—anywhere from $10,000 to above $100,000. The reasons for the high costs remain ambiguous and may be driven by financial interests rather than by costs or techniques.

In summary, bone marrow derived stem cells have enormous potential and are the mainstay for current research initiatives.

4.6 Adipose Tissue Derived Stem Cells

Several scientists and doctors recommend using adipose tissue derived stem cells instead of bone marrow derived cells. Until recently, bone marrow was perceived as the only significant reservoir of stem cells in the body. However, other—perhaps even more abundant—sources are now recognized, including adipose tissue. Subcutaneous fat is readily available in most patients and can easily be harvested in ample amounts. Therefore, adipose derived stem cells, also known as the stromal vascular fraction, can easily be isolated in therapeutically relevant amounts from fat tissue. This isolation can be performed in a matter of hours by simple enzymatic tissue digestion and centrifugation, which eliminates the need for cultivation and expansion.

This renders adipose tissue derived stem cells as a possible candidate for autologous (from the same patient) stem cell transplantation in the acute phase of certain diseases, including heart attacks. To date, adipose tissue derived stem cells have been used with a wide variety of diseases, including systemic sclerosis, osteoarthritis, and complex wound repair (including partial mastectomy defects after breast cancer).[14]

To use adipose derived stem cells from the patient (to be reinjected after isolation) does require a small surgical procedure to retrieve the cells from fat tissue. A mini liposuction is performed in order to aspirate enough fat tissue, usually from the belly fat using a long aspiration catheter through a few pin holes in the stomach, local anesthetics, and an anesthetic fluid through the catheter. In experienced hands, this approach is a routine procedure that easily can be performed in about twenty minutes. Some researchers believe that the output of stem cells from adipose tissue preparations yields a hundredfold more cells than retrieval from a bone marrow aspirate. The FDA, however, has not favored adipose derived cell injections (even autologous), and still has not approved them. The FDA has issued warnings more than once against centers and doctors who use this approach in light of possible manipulation of the cells after retrieval.

In fact, one of the main training centers for stem cell therapy in the US (based in Florida) has promoted adipose derived stem cells for years, but that center has received several warning letters from the FDA as well as cease-and-desist orders for irregularities in the handling of the tissues. More and more physicians are now shying away from using adipose derived cells mainly for this reason.

As in the above sources, costs vary. *CBC Canada* shared that the cost of stem cell therapy is $5,000 to $8,000 per stem cell treatment for the Cell Surgical Network (CSN) following its protocol to collect fat tissue and process it before reinjecting it directly or intravenously into the same patient. And according to an analysis of the company BioInformant, the cost of stem cell therapy ranges from less than $5,000 to more than $25,000. In general, orthopedic treatments are less expensive, while treatments for chronic and complex conditions are more expensive.

In general, adipose tissue derived stem cells have potential but are unlikely to be advantageous over the future role of bone marrow derived or allogenic stem cells and are less likely to be FDA-approved in the foreseeable future.

4.7 Myocyte Derived Stem Cells

One of the first studied stem cell therapies used myoblasts or muscle tissue derived stem cells that were obtained using a muscle biopsy (usually from the leg muscles). These myoblast stem cells were used in the so-called MARVEL trial in patients with heart disease, which showed some improvements in a six-minute walk test after the procedure as well as in a few other studies.[15]

Currently, myocyte derived stem cells are not used in clinical stem cell therapy, most likely because of the more complicated processes of skeletal muscle biopsy and preparing the tissue to isolate the myoblasts. This is less efficient than bone marrow or adipose derived stem cells.

4.8 Menstrual Blood Derived Stem Cells

Menstrual blood contains mesenchymal stem cells. These cells have attracted a great deal of attention due to their exceptional advantages, including easy access, frequently accessible sample source, and no need for complex ethical and surgical interventions, as compared to other tissues.

Menstrual blood derived stem cells possess all the major stem cell properties and even have a greater proliferation and differentiation potential than bone marrow derived cells, making them a potential tool in a further clinical practice. The potential of menstrual blood stem cells to differentiate into a large variety of tissue cells has been investigated in some studies, but those studies used small numbers of patients.

No data is available about current costs or charges for using menstrual blood cells derived stem cell therapies, but costs should be lower than bone marrow derived or adipose tissue derived stem cell preparations.

Although a very limited number of studies have been done, the menstrual blood derived stem cells might emerge as an efficient and easily accessible source of multipotent cells for one and joint cartilage engineering and cell-based, joint-protective therapies.

4.9 Placenta Tissue Derived Stem Cells

The human term placenta is a prime candidate for a stem cell source, as it is available in nearly unlimited supply, ethically problem-free, and easily procured. Placental cells display differentiation capacity toward all three germ layers while also displaying immunomodulatory effects, therefore supporting the possibility that they could be applied in an allogeneic transplantation setting. Although promising data has been reported to date, further study is required to fully characterize the differentiation potential of placenta derived cells and to identify their possible clinical applications.

There are several aspects of placenta derived stem cells that make them more attractive as cellular therapy than their counterparts from other tissues, such as cells from bone marrow or adipose tissue in regenerative medicine. Placenta derived stem cells have been used to treat a variety of disorders, such as cancer, liver, and cardiac diseases, ulcers, bone repair, and neurological diseases. Placenta derived stem cells are a relatively newly recognized type of cell with specific immunomodulatory properties. Its mechanisms are still unknown. Placenta derived stem cells secrete some soluble factors that seem to be responsible for their therapeutic effects, i.e., they have paracrine effects. But they can also serve as cellular vehicles and/or delivery systems for medications due to their migration capacity and their ability to be attracted to injury sites.[16]

Nanotechnology is an important field that has undergone rapid development in recent years for the treatment of injured organs. Due to the special characteristics of placenta derived stem cells, the combination of these cells with nanotechnology is a significant and highly promising field that could provide significant contributions to the regenerative medicine field in the near future.

Per definition, if placenta derived stem cells are used in a person other than the woman the placenta comes from, those cells are allogenic. Stem cells can be isolated from two regions of the placenta: the amniotic mesenchyme and the chorionic mesenchyme. Cells isolated from these placental regions should be confirmed to be of fetal origin. For practical purposes, the stem cells are defined by three criteria: adherence to plastic, expression of specific antigens, and their ability to differentiate into certain cell types.

More than 95 percent of the placenta derived stem cell population must express certain (measurable) tissue markers, such as CD73, CD105, and CD90, while other markers should be less expressed. Different regions of the placenta can give rise to different types of placenta derived stem cell populations, but a dive into these differences is far beyond the frame of this overview.

To harvest stem cells from the human term placenta, umbilical cord blood is first allowed to drain from the placenta, which is then dissected carefully. Two different approaches are used to isolate stem cells. In the first approach, placental fetal membranes are manually separated from each other, then either the amnion or the chorion is enzymatically degraded using different concentrations of digestive enzymes such as trypsin, dispase, and collagenase. Pellets of placental stem cells recovered after centrifugation are then plated on culture dishes in a standard culture medium. Placental stem cells are then identified by their adherence to the culture dish and expression of specific surface markers. The second approach differs from the first in that no prior membrane separation is performed. The entire placental tissue is dissected and enzymatically digested.

While there is no reliable information about current costs for placenta derived stem cell therapies, apparently providers charge based on the amount of isolated and injected cells, and it can cost between $3,000 and $10,000 per treatment.

Regardless of their isolation technique, studies have shown that placenta derived stem cells are actively involved in immunosuppression and have comparable characteristics to other sources of stem cells, such as those derived from bone marrow.

4.10 Umbilical Cord Stem Cells and Wharton's Jelly

In placental mammals, the umbilical cord is a structure that connects the placenta to the developing fetus, thereby providing a source of fetal nourishment. In humans, it is forty to sixty centimeters long at term with a girth of one to two centimeters. The structure appears simple with a single outer layer of amniotic epithelium that encloses a mucoid connective tissue through which three vessels, a vein and two arteries, carry oxygenated and deoxygenated blood between the placenta and fetus, respectively. Unlike other vessels of similar diameter in the human, the umbilical vessels have only two (not three) vessel wall layers. The role of the third protective layer in other blood vessels, however, is fulfilled by slimy connective tissue. This layer is called "Wharton's Jelly" after it was first described by Thomas Wharton in 1656. The slimy layer also prevents kinking of the vessels with movement of the fetus in the womb, although Wharton thought that the jelly served as a surrogate lymph transport system. The jelly contains no other blood or lymph vessels and is not innervated.

Human umbilical cord is a promising source for mesenchymal stem cell retrieval. The collection is painless and uses otherwise discarded tissues (medical waste) without any ethical concerns. These cells have shown the ability to differentiate into three germ layers, accumulate in damaged tissue or inflamed regions, promote tissue repair, and modulate immune response. There are different protocols in place for the retrieval and isolation of umbilical cord blood derived stem cells from the various compartments of the umbilical blood—Wharton's Jelly, veins, arteries, the endothelial cell lining, and regions outside the blood vessels (perivascular regions).

Umbilical cord derived stem cells have a distinct capacity for self-renewal while maintaining their multipotency, i.e., the ability to differentiate into different cell types, although some differentiation abilities might be incomplete.

While embryonic stem cells likely possess the most potent source for any reparative, regenerative, or tissue-engineering mechanisms, their use is limited by ethical concerns, lack of any legal regulations to protect the embryonic tissue, and limitations of technical difficulties with the depletion of immature cells that may result in the formation of tumors (teratoma).

Umbilical cord derived stem cells are pluripotent in nature. The umbilical cord derived stem cells have attracted great interest because of their immunomodulatory properties. Umbilical cord derived stem cells are the most promising tools for regenerative medicine and immunotherapy.

4.11 Cardiac Derived Stem Cells and Cardiospheres

The first reported stem cells in the heart were identified and isolated based on the expression of certain stem cell factor receptors, in particular CD117 or c-kit. Stem cells are identified by their expression of certain receptors. Cardiac derived stem cells are multipotent, self-renewing, and capable of forming heart muscle cells, smooth muscle cells, and vascular cells.[17]

In the adult heart, most of the cardiac derived stem cells reside in the atrium and the ventricular apex, but, overall, they are found in low numbers in the heart. These cells can be isolated and cultured over long-term periods without losing their self-renewing capacity and without showing evidence of senescent growth arrest or significant aging.

Some clinical trials have used cardiac derived stem cell infusion in patients with heart failure and have showed that intracoronary administration of these cells improved the heart's strength (left ventricular ejection fraction) and reduced the area of damaged tissue.[18]

Spherical aggregates of cells grown from heart biopsies are called cardiospheres. These conglomerations of cell mixtures can provide a source for cardiac derived stem cells in the experimental laboratory. I have been personally involved in clinical studies using these cell preparations for patients with heart attacks and congestive heart failure.[19]

Some of the clinical studies involving cardiac derived stem cells and cardiospheres have been finalized and published, while others are underway. A major break-through for its role in cardiac repair in real human patients, however, has not been established yet.

4.12 Somatic Cell Nuclear Transfer (SCNT)

The idea behind somatic cell nuclear transfer (SCNT) was to generate an individual's personalized embryonic stem cells from that same person's somatic cells. In other words, it is a laboratory method of creating an embryo from a body cell combined with an egg cell, which is used in reproductive cloning procedures. There are several ethical issues with this method, including the fact that embryos are manipulated, which could cause possible physical harm in the developing embryo. The creation of human beings in a laboratory, of course, has several ethical, moral, and religious objections and at the current time is far beyond what any physician would consider to be a viable treatment option for any disease. The method was very controversially discussed in the media when one individual tried to clone himself in order to gain immortality. This individual stated in front of news cameras during a CNN report in 2014 while holding a Petri dish, "This in the Petri dish is me before I was born." It appears obvious that somatic cell nuclear cloning of human beings or the creation of embryonic cells for stem cell therapies is not—and should not—be permitted at this time and raises several ethical concerns.

5

The Search for Something New

For centuries—if not thousands of years or from the beginning of human life—experience has taught us to recognize a difference in physical capabilities as a function of time. Time in this sense represents the biological development from in-utero cellular division following conception to cellular specialization to organ development by birth, which is followed by fine-tuning our organic function with growth and differentiation. The clumsy hand and leg movements of a newborn are nondirected and years away from the motor skills of a classical musician hammering Chopin etudes down the piano.

As teenagers and young adults, we often feel strong, infallible, and invincible without any realistic sense of the progressive weakness our muscles and organs surely go through over years and decades, finally leading to frailty in old age.

Isn't it amazing that, despite all the advances in technology and modern medicine, we have not found the cure for aging yet?

Well, the process of getting older does not need to be something bad, as long as we can continue to function as more or less independent human beings. The connotation of getting older, however, is the development of chronic diseases, especially those caused by degeneration. Keep in mind that the majority of illnesses stem from one of four mechanisms (the "pathological quadro"):

1. Inflammation (as a result of infection or trauma)
2. Lack of oxygen (as in calcification of arteries, diabetes, heart diseases)
3. Biological degeneration (as caused by joint arthritis, back pain, dementia)
4. Malignant mutation (as in all cancers)

Once we understand that all diseases, especially those occurring with advanced age, are caused by any of the above pathophysiologic or pathological quartet, we understand that future therapies must address all of those conditions in order to fight age-associated diseases.

Medicine has made major advances, especially in the last century. Remember that just one hundred years ago, the majority of people died of infectious diseases, such as tuberculosis, diphtheria, and the plaque. In the 1900s, approximately 110,000 people died each year from tuberculosis. The identification of bacteria as the source of many of those diseases changed the world of medicine tremendously. The German physician Robert Koch is credited as one of the creators of bacteriology and microbiology from studying the diseases anthrax, cholera, and tuberculosis.

Louis Pasteur then developed the first vaccines against anthrax, cholera, and rabies in the late nineteenth century by using weakened microbes that did not cause disease but created immunization against it upon further exposure. For example, in 2017, 9,105 cases of tuberculosis were reported in the US, which represents a decline of 1.6 percent from the year before. Even though tuberculosis is still a major health problem worldwide because of its high prevalence in developing countries, it can now be successfully treated in most cases. Likewise, HIV and AIDS became a worldwide epidemic in the nineties, even though sporadic cases were reported in the seventies (but not named as such since no definite diagnosis could be made). In 1983 and 1984, the Pasteur Institute in France and the National Cancer Institute in the US found the virus that caused AIDS. The virus resulted in a reduction of the immune system with resultant infections and malignancies. AIDS is still somewhat incurable, but the mortality has dramatically decreased from approximately 1.95 million deaths at its peak in 2005/2006 to less than one million in 2017 with the availability of retroviral combination therapy that has clearly been shown to prolong life.

As the number of death cases secondary to infections went down, the prevalence of death from chronic degenerative diseases went up dramatically. As a result of aging, approximately 100,000 people die each day. The majority of these cases are due to cardiovascular diseases such as coronary artery disease, stroke, heart attack, peripheral artery disease, and generalized atherosclerosis. Today, heart and vascular problems are the number one killer worldwide. Despite many advances in drug therapy and surgical treatment options over the last few decades, heart diseases—especially blockages of the blood vessels in the heart and congestive heart failure—remain the leading cause of death for women and men in the Western world.

Due to more early recognition of what we call "typical symptoms" of heart problems, such as chest pain or breathing problems, and broader education for the public about these signs and symptoms, the possibilities for treating heart attacks or unstable angina have improved dramatically. Now we usually perform a cardiac catheterization if a patient comes to the hospital with signs and symptoms of a heart attack, which means we insert a small catheter either through the groin or through the arm to the heart to visualize potential blockages in the arteries. If a blocked artery is detected, a balloon angioplasty can be performed, i.e., widening the blocked artery and inserting a metal ring (stent) to keep the artery open.

Stent in Coronary Artery

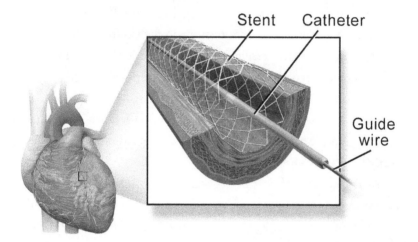

These procedures paired with modern drug therapy have significantly improved the outcomes of patients who suffer a heart attack and have dramatically reduced mortality. Furthermore, the recognition and aggressive treatment of risk factors contributing to heart attacks, such as smoking, diabetes, high blood pressure, and high cholesterol, have also reduced the overall prevalence of heart attacks. Since more and more patients now survive heart attacks compared to previous decades, there is also a growing prevalence of chronic heart diseases, in particular congestive heart failure.

The older people become—and the longer people live—the higher their chances are of developing heart failure. Especially with the aging baby boomer generation, more patients than ever before will be flooding doctors' offices in the coming decades because of chronic cardiovascular diseases. At this point, heart failure cannot be cured. It is, in most cases, a result of irreversible damage of heart muscle cells, which is either caused by lack of oxygen, inflammation, or degeneration, among other causes. Despite the advances in technology for early diagnostics and treatment using medications like beta blockers, angiotensin converting enzymes inhibitors, angiotensin receptor blockers, or the implantation of pacemaker defibrillators in addition to lifestyle changes such as weight loss, moderate exercise, and adherence to medication regimens or fluid intake restrictions, patients with chronic congestive heart failure are frequent flyers in hospitals because of volume overload leading to shortness of breath and/or water accumulation, such as edema in the lungs, legs, or anywhere else in the body.

In the last thirty years, very few new medications were developed to treat these conditions. The only quasi cure for congestive heart failure is a heart transplant. However, there are more than six million people in the US currently suffering from heart failure. There are approximately 150,000 newly diagnosed cases each year, but there are only 2,200 heart transplantations performed yearly in the US. That means that the majority of patients will not be candidates for a heart transplant.

There are several reasons patients might not qualify for a heart transplant. Among other reasons, this procedure requires the absence of significant comorbidities, appropriate compliance, appropriate insurance coverage, a caregiver plan provided by the patient, and age parameters (heart transplants are harder to perform in patients above seventy-five years of age). That means the vast majority of patients rely on medical therapy without any options for cure, and often there are only slight symptom improvements for a limited period of time while the disease progresses and finally leads to death. Newer surgical options, such as the insertion of a left or right ventricular pump device or even the implantation of a total artificial heart, can prolong life and improve symptoms. These are either used as a bridge to transplantation or what we call "destination therapy," meaning they stay in forever. However, these surgical options remain the last resort for only a very limited number of patients.

There is an enormous need to research technologies that can replace damaged tissue in the heart with functioning heart muscle cells, thus improving the strength of weak hearts. Regenerative therapy aims to solve this issue by attempting to use stem cells, growth factors, or gene therapy to help the body heal itself—at least to a certain degree. Heart failure is (thankfully) a great research subject since it is abundant, easy to study, and, so far, nobody has found a cure for it.

Similarly, there are other conditions leading to chronic debilitating changes in many organ systems. Diabetes is one of them. In type 1 or juvenile diabetes, the pancreas does not produce enough insulin to counteract the effects of sugar in the body. These young patients require daily insulin injections from an early age and continue for the rest of their lives. The treatment aims to maintain normal blood sugar levels, avoiding diabetes-related changes in all other organs. Diabetes can cause diseases of the eyes, the kidneys, the heart, the brain, and the entire vascular system. This condition cannot be cured as of today, either.

Type 2 diabetes, on the other hand, is adult-onset elevated sugar levels, and it affects more than thirty million patients in the US. Type 2 diabetes also causes blindness, kidney failure, heart attacks, strokes, peripheral vascular disease, and nerve damage. Treatment includes diet and exercise, as well as medication to lower blood sugar and sometimes insulin substitution.

Despite these treatments, which certainly have improved the outcomes and complications of diabetes, the objective of reducing vascular complications has not been met sufficiently to date. Therefore, new treatments are required to avoid the long-term deadly consequences of conditions such as diabetes, high blood pressure, or congestive heart failure. The challenge for regenerative medicine is to focus more on the underlying causes that lead to the symptoms instead of focusing on pure symptom relief. The task of modern medicine is to diagnose diseases much earlier, even before symptoms are apparent. Furthermore, we should try to replenish damaged materials in our bodies. In other words, we need to find ways to regrow organs in a Petri dish and help our bodies repair themselves.

Regenerative medicine in its simplest form would mean to exchange damaged or dead cells with juvenile functioning cells. The whole idea behind stem cell therapy is to help stem cells develop into fully functional mature cells in whatever organ needs them. However, that the simple injection of cellular suspension into a damaged heart can completely restore cardiac function in a patient with heart failure is still more wishful thinking than reality. On the other hand, many studies have shown that the addition of stem cell injections have improved outcomes for healing wounds, skin ulcers, and improvement of organ function in preliminary small human and animal studies.

Still, much more research is needed.

As I mentioned before, for heart failure, the ultimate therapy would be heart transplantation. But one of the reasons for the relatively low number of heart transplants performed worldwide is the lack of donor organs. Hearts are not available from the shelves; someone has to die for a suitable heart to save another person's life. The organ shortage creates relatively long waiting lists, even for patients who have been eligible for heart transplantation for many months or even years. According to several publications, approximately 30 percent of patients die while on the waiting list. There is general agreement among physicians and researchers that much more needs to be done to help these patients.

And it all starts in the research labs with the brains of some smart people with oftentimes unconventional ideas.

It's amazing what can be done by researchers nowadays. For example, whole organs can now be created by 3-D printing mechanisms, where the "ink" is made of cells printed on a prepared scaffold with special 3-D bioprinters to build a living organ. According to some of the biotech leaders in the field, bioprinted skin could be just a few years away, and complex organs such as hearts, livers, and kidneys maybe less than a decade away.

More studies are needed to develop bioprinting and advanced regenerative medicine in order to successfully achieve a paradigm shift in modern medicine to treating the underlying problem rather than covering up the symptoms.

6

The Unknown and My Personal Doubts

When I first heard about people performing stem cell therapy, I couldn't believe it. In fact, I could not believe that some healthcare providers would perform any unapproved therapies in their offices without participating in a clinical study or publishing a scientific paper in a peer-reviewed journal on the subject.

Maybe it was my European thinking but growing up in the academic world of a prestigious high-tech university in Germany (Rheinisch-West-faelische Technische Hochschule RWTH, University of Technology Aachen), as well as the prestigious University of Vienna (Universitaet Wien), my colleagues and I were taught with quite a different scientific mindset back then.

6.1 The Experts

The European philosophy was that if you are a scientist and physician and plan to recommend or perform any novel therapeutic approach, you must do the necessary basic research work over many years. You would have studied cell cultures during long nights in the lab, you would have conducted tons of experimental animal studies, you would have created safety and tolerability studies in human volunteers, participated in landmark clinical trials in real patients, and then you would have published all of the data in peer-reviewed international scientific journals.

Then and only then, you might have gained the reputation amongst your peers as an *expert* in this particular field. Once you are considered an expert, you might have the appropriate expertise and knowledge to talk about and perform novel technologies and therapies based on your years of hard work and experience.

Well, this European academic mindset obviously doesn't carry over to the US, which is sometimes good and other times bad.

I remember the first time I was invited to attend a sponsored dinner lecture in Texas. I had just been appointed as Professor of Medicine at the historic and highly recognized University of Texas Medical Branch (UTMB) in Galveston, Texas, and even though I usually do not attend this kind of dinner lecture (unless I am the speaker), I went to familiarize myself with my new environment and colleagues. The doctor who gave the lecture was an assistant professor at the university, and he talked about statin therapy (lipid lowering drugs) and its benefits on cardiovascular health.

The lecturer was actually a very pleasant guy and good clinical physician, as I learned later; however, he had never participated in any of the major clinical trials, he had never done research on statins himself, and he had never published any scientific manuscripts on statin therapy.

Somewhat confused by these facts, I initially thought, "Why in the world would I even listen to this guy's lecture? He himself knows as much as the audience about statins but is giving a lecture about it to other physicians. What the heck?"

To top it off, he used slides prepared by the pharmaceutical company that manufactured a particular statin. These slides were approved by the FDA to be used in commercial talks. Moreover, the guy was paid somewhere around $1,000 for giving the lecture by the drug company.

I could not believe the whole concept, and that was my first "academic" experience working as a clinical doctor in the US in 2003.

Again, in Europe, I would have not seen anything like that. If someone gives a lecture about statins, you can be sure that this person is a real expert in the field, that they have been part of the major clinical studies, and they know much more than the audience about the topic. This is why someone would be invited to give a lecture and why academic scholars would attend to it to get the inside scoop on the topic.

Similarly, years later, I heard about an orthopedic surgeon who uses stem cell therapy for arthritis and other joint conditions. I knew the guy to be a nice fellow, but he had never published a scientific paper about stem cells nor done basic experimental work. He still marketed himself as the expert, and I started thinking, "This must be a joke."

Another physician I came across shortly thereafter was even worse—a dermatologist who treated foreign patients with chronic severe heart diseases using stem cells and charged them tens of thousands of dollars in cash for it. He actually treated a patient with severe end-stage heart failure with an intravenous injection of stem cells and claimed to be an expert in this field. He had no clue how to treat a patient with heart failure in general and offered "advanced treatment options" for end-stage heart failure.

I could not believe my eyes and ears.

Not surprisingly, these two physicians did not have admitting or consulting privileges in any prestigious hospital, they did not have any academic appointments at a university, and they had neither regional, national, nor international reputation as scientists or clinicians. They both did, however, have good marketing strategies for how to create a lucrative business. Naturally, they never presented any follow-up data at any scientific conference, since they had none, and I must assume that they did not care much about long-term outcomes.

Again, both of these physicians are still practicing and appear to be successful in their business endeavors. How do they get patients to believe their unsubstantiated claims of being experts in the field of stem cell therapy? I still do not understand. Maybe they have enough fake reviews on their websites that potential patients read and are convinced by, but these reviews have no meaning with regard to a clinical or scientific expertise or quality of care by any physician. They represent a personal experience of a few patients about how they felt being treated in the physicians' offices, similar to reviews hospitals received in the past. Traditionally, bad hospital reviews were often based on the taste of the hospital food rather than on any medical quality of care. But how should potential future patients know this? How can a patient trust a physician and get objective data regarding their quality of work? The answer is not reading consumer reviews on the web, but patients then often rely on marketed claims when no objective information is made available (which would be devastating for many).

6.2 My Experiment

In a recent experiment, I asked a friend of mine who had nothing to do with our medical business and is a prospective patient to call different agencies and physician practices in the greater Los Angeles area that marketed stem cell therapies for different clinical conditions. During the calls, he stated that he had hip pain and was offered hip replacement surgery because of the diagnosis of aseptic hip necrosis that occurred after a skiing accident over one year ago. He randomly called five clinics offering stem cell therapies for joint problems to get some basic information about stem cell therapy based on their website marketing for the treatment of hip arthritis and pain. He asked the following questions:

1. What types of cells are used?
2. Where are the cells coming from?
3. What are the expected clinical results?
4. How many patients have been treated with this condition in your practice?

He also particularly asked about the antigenic potential of allogenic stem cells.

No sufficiently clear answers were received from any of the five clinics. The clinic representatives were salespeople who had no understanding of what he was asking for. Five out of five clinics stated that they have excellent results but did not provide the number of patients treated. Five out five clinics also stated that their cells are safe and claimed no side effects would occur. All five clinics stated that they had never heard about any antigenic potential with their stem cell treatment (and did not even know what that meant). No one provided specific responses to any of the questions. They all, however, offered payment plans for the reimbursement of the treatment.

After hearing about these and other experiences of people close to me, I felt like it was all nonsense without any scientific evidence. I had no intention to be part of this kind of treatment nor be named in context with this level of clinics and practitioners. However, these clinics do have followers, meaning that something about whatever they do must work well, even though they have no real pathophysiologic or biochemical understanding of it. But is that not how evidence-based medicine works? We may not know why something works, but as long as it helps patients, who cares?

In medicine, we do many things when we have no clue how and why they work. For example, one of the most well-known phenomena is that no one knows how anesthetics such as *propofol* work, but every anesthesiologist in the world uses it. Similarly, we don't know how stem cells work successfully to treat chronic pain, but thousands of patients and doctors swear on their efficacy.

Anyhow, I was very skeptical to believe any of the anecdotal reports or the nice-looking case studies presented at age-management conferences. I have been presenting scientific studies at international conferences regularly since my very first presentation at one of the American Heart Association conferences in 1989, and I know very well which data is presented—and which is not. In the mind of a researcher used to a systematic approach to a scientific question, there is no real evidence of a treatment's efficacy unless it has been demonstrated in double-blind, placebo-controlled, randomized, large-scale trials conducted by reliable investigators in reputable academic institutions. And, if that is the case, only then do the professional societies adapt the study's data and add it with recommendations into treatment guidelines that are the basis for medical practice in the US and all over the world.

6.3 How Do Ideas Become Standard Therapy?

Once a novel therapy has been adapted into professional society guidelines, insurance companies accept it and its costs years later, at least in part, and it becomes part of a normal treatment regimen for the public. The process for that is much more complicated than outlined here, but the basic principle is as described.

The level of recommendations in different guidelines (for example, the guidelines for the management of heart failure in an adult by the American Heart Association/American College of Cardiology and the European Society of Cardiology and The Heart Failure Society of America) is dependent on the level of evidence, whether the treatment recommendations are supported by large-scale trials or by consensus from experts in the field. In order to come to this point, however, randomized trials need to be conducted. These trials and studies must undergo a peer-reviewed process before publication in a scientific journal, then experts from the above societies gather to write the guidelines or adapt the current guidelines, which then will be published and become standard recommendations.

Coming back to the anecdotal success stories of single stem cell injections, they did not impress me at all. I was actually more impressed by how well some physicians presented completely unreproducible cases and the effect their talk had on other physicians in the audience. I felt like I was in Ancient Rome in midst of "*panem et circenses,*" which means "*bread and games,*" i.e., entertaining the masses like a show in Las Vegas. Perhaps that was the intent in the first place and was the reason the conferences were held in Las Vegas. That sort of presentation does work well—at least for a while.

6.4 The KISS Technique

In order to process scientifically, I decided to think through the stem cell technical idea in a more or less systemic fashion. That is, I chose to use the *KISS* technique (as one of my professors taught me years ago). The KISS technique in research comes from the fact that any scientific study becomes complicated through its course and analysis; therefore, it is essential to use KISS in the initial study design, which stands for "*Keep It Simple Stupid.*" The study design has to be simple, and the study has follow through without any violation of the protocol. The study hypothesis also has to be simple. Ideally it should be a question that can be answered by "Yes" or "No." For example, does drug A reduce the size of a heart attack in diabetic patients? In this type of a study, a working hypothesis or question has to be formulated, and the study design is created to answer that single question with simply "Yes" or "No." Then you keep in mind that the study results will tell you if drug A reduced the size of heart attacks in diabetic patients in the study if it is given at the time written in the study protocol for the population subtype written in the study protocol—and nothing besides that.

The study data, however, is often extrapolated into larger, unstudied populations, which itself might lead to follow-up studies, confirmatory studies, or studies showing contradicting results. That is how clinical research works and how it is usually conducted.

Therefore, in the case of regenerative cell effects, we created simple study designs using one type of cells to test one hypothesis in one specific animal model. Without going into too much detail of an example, which would be beyond the frame of this publication, we were the first to demonstrate that embryonic heart muscle cells do survive if implanted in host heart tissue in rats that had heart attacks.[20] Furthermore, the cell injections did, in fact, reduce the amount of damaged tissue as measured by a reduction in infarcts sizes.

6.5 My Basic Research

For the sake of providing just a brief idea of my research, I skip over several years of further experimental animal studies using different types of embryonic cells, stem cells, and growth factors in different laboratory settings between the Max Planck Institute for Experimental and Physiologic Cardiology in Bad Nauheim in Germany (where I received a scholarship from the German Heart Foundation working under Professor Dr. Wolfgang Schaper), the Heart Research Institute at the University of Southern California in Los Angeles, working under Professor Dr. Robert Kloner sponsored by an NIH grant, and the Rheinisch Westfaelische Technische Hochschule (RWTH University of Technology) in Aachen, Germany, working under Professor Dr. Peter Hanrath, as well as in my own laboratories.

Only after doing tons of basic research experiments using different cell types in different models, I slowly started realizing that the hypothetical regenerative potential of stem cells might translate into clinical medicine, meaning there might be a huge clinical potential of this kind of therapy working for real patients and resulting in clinical improvements for different conditions. Even though I performed tons of basic research experiments, I am, by nature, a clinical doctor dealing with patients, their symptoms, degeneration of tissue, loss of function, and loss of lives on a daily basis. Seeing the amazing results of stem cell injections on different pathophysiologic mechanisms and their reparative potential in the experimental setting was an eye-opener, and I could not wait to get my hands on clinical studies with real patients.

After gaining basic research data and our initial clinical experience (which was done outside the US at a time when no one in the country could do stem cell research in humans for regulatory and ethical reasons), we did participate in large-scale multicenter trials using stem cells. Thereafter, we created or own clinical studies, which we are still conducting up to this day. These studies may or may not be placebo-controlled in order to allow all participating patients to receive the benefits of the powerful cells within the frame of the clinical studies.

Today, I am a strong believer and supporter of stem cell therapy and do see it as the future of medicine. But the way cells are used is dependent on the background and experience of the investigators and, in today's world, cannot be generalized and deserve differentiation and quality control. Their use is spreading, especially among those who can afford it. Have you ever wondered why some of the most well-known celebrities look so great for their age? They use stem cells. I would never reveal the names of any of our patients, nor would I ever release anyone's protected health information, but I can assure you that we have treated many people you would recognize—with great success, as recognizable in their improved health and young appearance.

7.

Aging and Anti-Aging Medicine

T he term "anti-aging medicine" has been popularized in the last fifteen years but has been criticized heavily by the academic establishment. In fact, the term was recently banned in the media since it can mislead consumers and foster wrong expectations. Several years ago, I was actually invited to give a lecture during an anti-aging medicine conference, which I did not take very seriously at the time.

As a researcher and scientist, I used to give lectures and present my group's latest scientific data annually at the world's largest cardiology conferences, such as the annual conferences for the American Heart Association, the American College of Cardiology, and the European Society of Cardiology, with 40,000 to 60,000 participants from around the world in attendance. It was a must for young investigators working at a prestigious German university hospital to have a presence on the international stage with competitive scientists; otherwise, we were considered academic nobodies.

There was no question that we all submitted our scientific results in abstract form to the conferences, hoping that at least some would be accepted for presentation. It always worked out that most of us entered the world of established scientists with an international reputation in our fields within a few years.

Coming from that background, I did not take this first "anti-aging medicine" conference seriously. However, at that point in my busy life as a clinical cardiologist, I thought any one-to-two-day break to give a lecture was at least a way to get out of the daily routine, get on a plane, and turn off my phone, at least for a few hours. When I arrived at the conference, which was held in Las Vegas, and glanced through the scientific program, I did not recognize the names of any of the presenters. There was nobody I was used to being around from prestigious institutions such as Harvard, Yale, Oxford, Stanford, Tokyo, Vienna, USC, or UCLA (where I was from).

When it came to the actual lectures, I was not surprised to find mediocre scientific class, poor data presentations, and mostly anecdotal points with no clinical or research importance in my mind. In contrast, I thought the lecture I gave was excellent—at least in comparison to other presentations. While I found the whole conference somewhat scientifically unprofessional, I did wonder how some presenters were able to speak so well and skillfully sell their nonscientific data to an audience composed of physicians. Plus, I was somewhat impressed by how some of these physicians were using nonapproved and alternative methods to treat their patients. Further, I was impressed by the individual results, even those from using supplements that made a difference in people's symptoms. It was not scientific, but it was still impressive.

The following year, I was invited back to that same conference. I showed up and presented my scientific lecture, but this time to a much larger audience than the year before. I couldn't believe my eyes. While 150 physicians attended the meeting the year before, more than 600 doctors were in the lecture halls this second year—doctors for internal medicine, plastic surgery, cardiology, and orthopedic surgery, among many other specialties.

I talked to many of the attendees to find out why they were there. There appeared to be two main reasons why more and more physicians were attending these kinds of conferences:

1. To add an instrument to their medical practice, offering "anti-aging medicine" as a means to increase their revenue; or
2. To learn how to stay younger themselves since most of them were middle-aged baby boomers who feared the odds of upcoming age-related diseases.

7.1 Anti-Aging Medicine

The anti-aging idea was further popularized by individuals such as Dr. Jeffrey Life, a general practitioner from Las Vegas who became the face of the company Cenegenics. Cenegenics did not invent anything new for medicine but popularized the concept of physician-supervised exercise, nutrition, metabolism balance, and hormonal balance, especially by using injections of growth hormones and testosterone in men. The lifestyle changes and injections resulted in weight loss, increased muscle, increased energy, and increased stamina that made the seventy-year-old Jeffrey Life look like a thirty-year-old bodybuilder. The company became very successful and is now selling their programs in every city in the country.

While their business and marketing concept is extraordinary, many similar companies lack the scientific background and expertise to validate their anecdotal successes in a systematic and controllable fashion. However, the overall concept that exercise, lifestyle changes, improved nutrition, and possible replacement of certain vitamins and trace elements in the case of a demonstrated deficiency are beneficial in order to improve wellbeing is—without any doubts—of enormous clinical value, even though established academic institutions and leading clinical experts are not taking age-management practitioners seriously.

To be fair, neither did I at the beginning. It comes as no surprise that these approaches likely do support endogenous stem cell availability among the elderly and might even contribute to induction of mediator mechanisms.

In August of 2017, the fashion magazine *Allure* banned the term "anti-aging" with the intention of wiping it off the internet completely. The idea was that aging is a natural process to be embraced rather than fought against.

Even though aging is, in fact, something to honor and glorify rather than view as unattractive, the fact is that anti-aging efforts in medicine do not intend to abolish the validity of aging but rather delay the progression of age-related chronic degenerative diseases, which is an honorable effort. But the indiscriminate prescription of a growth hormone to every fifty-year-old man who wants to feel younger and sexier is medically unjustified, unethical, and even illegal. Plus, the long-term side effects are yet to be established. This is the kind of criticism that many of the anti-aging physicians are currently facing, and I do agree with that.

My advice is to stay away from the one-fits-all mentality some anti-aging providers try to sell since many of those providers do not have any scientific rationale to support their marketing claims. Also, take a look at the practitioners. Without any doubt, I can tell just walking through conferences who is injecting growth hormone and who is not. The growth hormone users have the classic acromegaly features—a huge forehead, huge chin, and enlarged tongue. They also develop enlargement of their heart (cardiomegaly) over time. I would stay away from those practitioners since they have obviously created a health problem for themselves they are not even aware of. Of course, I do not condemn all anti-aging physicians, but I do believe there are some who lack clinical or scientific reputation and market their services and products using false and unjustified claims.

Once again, aging is a beautiful thing but getting sick with age is not. Applying concepts commonly marketed as anti-aging medicine is not shameful as long as it is individualized, medically indicated, and physician-supervised on a regular basis. I do not think that this kind of anti-aging management should be banned, but it should be renamed as regenerative management. In fact, reasonable physicians would likely not use the term anti-aging at all but rather call it age management or age management medicine. Whatever it is called, regeneration of damaged tissue is the ideal focus for any medical management, even though natural regeneration was basically unknown in the armamentarium of physicians for the last 1,000 years.

7.2 The All-or-Nothing Phenomenon

In medical school, we as physicians learned about the *all-or-nothing phenomenon* in physiology. That simply means cells work if they are fueled by energy, usually in the form of adenosine triphosphate (ATP), which requires oxygen and nutrition. If nutrition is lacking, stored energy is used until it is depleted. If oxygen is lacking, ischemia (an inadequate blood supply) occurs with morphological and functional changes that start to happen immediately, i.e., within seconds. If ischemia lasts long enough, irreversible changes occur. Cell membranes rupture, which ultimately leads to necrosis (cell death), and that is usually followed by partial or total organ death. Death of a part of an organ (such as the heart) is followed by replacement fibrosis, which means replacement of formerly active heart muscle cells (cardiomyocytes) by inactive, collagen-based scar tissue without any metabolic or contractile function. There is no regeneration, especially not in the most important organs such as the heart and the brain.

That concept of *all-or-nothing* is what we were taught in medical school and what we all believed in. There are, however, conditions in which organs are smarter than we previously thought and switch reduced amounts of energy toward lifesaving mechanisms, keeping cell membranes intact at the cost of other functions. In the heart, this newly recognized phenomenon is called "hibernating myocardium." During hibernating myocardium, the heart acts *smart* and keeps its cells alive but does not pump well. This knowledge became the rationale for revascularization procedures such as coronary artery bypass surgery. It was shown that bypass surgery (as well as interventional revascularization strategies using percutaneous balloons) could be successful even in patients with weak hearts that formerly were thought to be too severely damaged.[21]

The concept of revascularizing weak, but not yet dead, tissue revolutionized vascular medicine but initially was heavily criticized, not lastly due to our studies, which were the first in the world to take biopsies from hibernating myocardium. These biopsies did not demonstrate the expected "normal tissue" but rather a progressive cellular degeneration with islands of scar tissue, contradicting the concept of an equilibrium of heart tissue with chronic lack of oxygen.[22] Our published data on the contrary showed that there is no steady state but a time-dependent "slow death." If—as shown in thousands of cases—for example, revascularization by coronary bypass surgery does restore weakened heart function over time, that would mean there is restoration of contractile elements or regeneration of dead tissue, against all odds of the all-or-nothing phenomenon. This only can be achieved with the recruitment of endogenous stem cells or, nowadays, by exogenous stem cell administration. Regeneration itself is mainly induced by stem cells; therefore, stem cell therapy should be in itself the mainstay of any age management or better-called "anti-disease management in the elderly" approach.

The real point of interest for any research, as well as for wishful thinking about anti-aging, is manyfold. For a long time, a human goal has been to prevent aging—the achievement of immortality. Though an intriguing concept, this idea touches religious beliefs as well as metaphysics. In many religions, the soul of an individual goes to heaven after the death of the body; therefore, the soul is immortal. There is, obviously, no living proof of this idea. In a theological context, we are reunited with the creator in a space outside of our visible and understandable world. The fact is our parents do live on in us and in our children after their earthly death. Thinking of our loved ones that passed away makes them somewhat living on in us. In a physical and metaphysical world, all life consists of energy and energy continues for eternity in the universe in one form or another, since energy cannot be created or destroyed and does not vanish.

As for medical advancements, there has been no major successful breakthrough in creating drugs or procedures that prevent aging in humans so far. On the other hand, research increasingly focuses on delaying the processes of aging. Several animal models have been successfully performed to increase the lifespan of mice up to 50 percent. By understanding the processes of aging, researchers try to target the components that lead to aging of cells, organs, and the entire human system.

7.3 Causes of Cellular Aging

These are many reasons why our cells, our organs, and our bodies age. Among others, some of the main pathophysiologic causes include:

1. Damage of DNA
2. Reduction of telomere length (on the chromosomes)
3. Accumulation of metabolic garbage within the cells and tissue
4. Buildup of senescent cells
5. Loss of blood vessel elasticity
6. Reduction of stem cell capacity and number
7. Mitochondrial damage
8. Reduction of proteins/histone production.

Efforts are underway in basic research labs, cell culture models, and animal models to address each of these causes with promising results, but only a few clinical studies have been performed in humans so far.

Besides the attempts to delay (rather than to prevent) aging, there is even more progress underway to reverse degeneration in aging. In other words, regenerative medicine—in particular, stem cell therapy—can, at least to some extent, replace dead cells and tissue and regenerate tissue morphology and function, thus repairing damage caused by aging. That, in fact, represents the most important advancement in modern medicine, which was unthinkable and unimaginable even just thirty years ago.

Think about it. Why do we care about aging? Isn't aging a natural biological process all living beings experience? Well, of course it is. But aging is not only a natural biological or physical process of change; aging is also the number-one cause of death in the world. According to an age-researching biologist, every single day, approximately 100,000 people die as a result of aging. Aging leads to death.

Moreover, aging is also the number-one risk factor for chronic degenerative diseases that ultimately lead to organ damage and death, such as cardiovascular disease (including heart attacks, heart failure, and strokes), diabetes (with resulting blindness, kidney failure, and loss of extremities), and cancer (with resulting organ damage, metastasis, and early death).

Aging is also the number-one risk factor for death. In contrast to other risks, such as obesity, uncontrolled hypertension, or bad diet habits, this risk factor cannot be manipulated by modern medicine—yet.

7.4 Medicine Today is Reactive

In today's world of medicine, we focus on symptom relief and prolonging life. For example, in my field of cardiology, I take patients to the cardiac catheterization laboratory every single day to perform coronary angiograms. I insert a plastic tube into people's groin or wrist and advance a catheter into the heart to visualize the blood vessels and evaluate whether there is a blockage that might create a life-threatening heart attack. If there is a blockage, I open it up and place a stent into the blood vessel to keep it from blocking again; thus, blood flow to the heart is improved. At the same time, I prescribe medicines to ease the chest pain patients experience if there is a blockage and give them blood thinners to prevent clotting in the arteries.

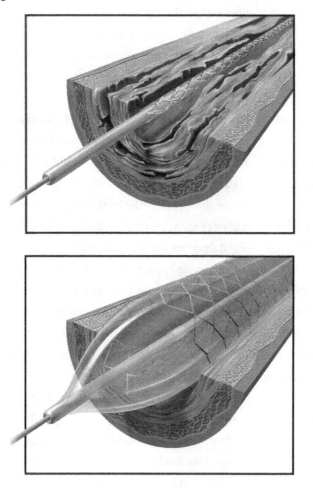

In other words, I am like a mechanic fixing a tube blocked by plaque. The plaque is caused by cholesterol calcifications, usually as a result of high blood pressure, diabetes, smoking, a strong family history of the same condition—and/or aging. For these reasons, we focus on therapies that help prevent calcifications. We treat diabetes with tablets or insulin, we treat elevated lipids with statins and other drugs, we give beta blockers and water pills with other things to reduce high blood pressure. These all have good, but oftentimes not sufficient, results. And we still do not address the main cause of all of this: aging.

Medicine still concentrates on symptoms like pain, fever, shortness of breath, or the inability to move an extremity because those are the reasons why patients usually come to see a doctor. We then prescribe medications to treat the symptoms, and we evaluate the cause by ordering several diagnostic tests. Too often, pain medications are prescribed by healthcare providers to help the relieve symptoms. The prescription pain medication epidemic, especially in the Western world, is caused by undifferentiated prescription practices, patient demand (nobody talks about that in the media yet), and the addictive properties of those drugs. The addictive properties are finally being looked at by regulatory agencies, which will hopefully help to reduce their use in the future. All drugs we use on a daily basis do have side effects, and they can result in damage, new symptoms, and sickness.

In addition, we use drugs that have been proven to have long-term benefits (such as aspirin in patients with strokes or documented coronary artery disease), reduce progression of the underlying disease (such as statins in patients with vascular calcifications), or improve survival (such as beta blockers and ACE inhibitors in patients with congestive heart failure). All of these measures come into place once the diseases are prominent and cause symptoms, and then we improve the status and delay further damage. But by this point, traditional medicine is way too late to reverse the disease. This kind of medicine is reactive. We react to symptoms and signs of disease that already exists.

In contrast, regenerative therapy (stem cell therapy) can now come into play since we have learned that we can reverse some damage (although we still cannot cure the diseases). Interestingly, this is not done at all in practice with the exception of ongoing clinical studies in large academic centers with very strict inclusion criteria by a very few clinician researchers who dare to try to provide patients with more than the standard options. The vast majority of physicians are still blind to the revolutionary idea of regeneration by stem cell use for obvious reasons but also for lack of better knowledge.

7.5 Thoughts on Regenerative Medicine

Not too long ago, I was approached by a patient. This patient was a lady in her late forties with a progressive musculoskeletal degenerative disease. Her muscles have gotten weaker in recent years, and there is no known cure for her condition so far.

Most patients with this condition end up in a wheelchair, and oftentimes on a respirator later since they are too weak to breathe on their own, and then they face early death. There are very few cases that demonstrate that stem cell therapy might reduce the speed of the progression of the disease (that theoretically could lead to some prolongation of life). But more importantly, stem cell injections have made patients feel subjectively better and stronger (as also shown in many other chronic incurable diseases such as heart failure).

So, this patient, in fact, came for a stem cell therapy consultation. She had problems with balance and walking for a prolonged period of time, a condition her father also experienced before he passed away prematurely. I explained the experimental nature in detail, the lack of large-scale clinical data, and the lack of FDA approval on this kind of treatment. The patient asked if I would use this treatment on my own sister if she was sick, and I responded, "Absolutely, there is nothing to lose in trying something new, outside the box, with a great promise."

In fact, at that time, we were conducting a clinical study free of charge to any patient in which we were testing a stem cell injection versus a placebo injection on symptom outcomes in this kind of condition. I told the patient that neither she or I would know whether she would receive the stem cell injection or the placebo but that only minor side effects would be expected from either injection. Further, due to the nature of the study, no guarantees could be given about whether the treatment would make any change in her symptoms since the outcome was unknown. The patient later asked her neurologist (who is not an academic neurologist) about participating in a stem cell therapy study and he told her, "I never would use stem cells, not even on my own child."

While I respect everyone's opinion, this person obviously did not consider anything outside the box to try to help a desperate patient in need of therapy when she could participate in a clinical study that might or might not help her.

There is nothing illegal or unethical about their opinion; it is just sad.

This patient never came back for any treatments or further opinions, and I heard that she now is completely bound to a wheelchair, unable to walk at all. This is a horrible but common story. I would never say that a stem cell therapy might have turned her fate around; however, it most likely would not have made things worse for her and might have had the potential to improve her condition temporarily. It might have improved her symptoms and her weakness somewhat or delayed the progression of her underlying deadly disease a bit. Why not try?

When the German F1 racing car world champion, Michael Schumacher, received a nondisclosed stem cell therapy from Professor Dr. Menasche in Paris in September of 2019, the famous British cardiologist Dr. Malhotra stated, "If it does not do harm, why not give it a try?"

But most healthcare providers do not share the same opinion so far, mainly based on a lack of convincing study data and knowledge.

7.6 Sick Care versus Healthcare

If we want to address the issues of aging that lead to chronic illnesses and death, we need to address aging itself rather than concentrating purely on medicine that is *reactive* to diseases. Medicine nowadays still represents more "sick care" rather than "healthcare." The few research efforts to combat the processes of aging only deal with improvement of function and morphology in order to improve quality of life by preventing or delaying the age-related diseases versus prolonging lifespan. This makes perfect sense from an ethical and economic point of view. If we have most people living to or past one hundred years old, we might create a population of progressive frailty and loss of decency with extreme high costs to any society. Instead, we should aim to improve functional capacity so that the elderly can live independently and work even into old age. Therefore, the goal is actually to extend "health span" rather than extending "life span."

In an ideal world, however, we should increase both health span and life span. If the current research in mice can prolong the life of rodents by 50 percent using certain types of gene therapy, theoretically we should be able to increase longevity in humans to live up to 120 years or more, as long as clinical studies support the safety, tolerance, and efficacy of such treatments.

This is the future, but it is not realistic as of today.

7.7 Blue Zones

If we look into research on aging in humans, there are certain environmental pockets in different parts of the world—from Japan to Sardinia to Loma Linda in California—with an abnormally large number of centenarians (people living beyond one hundred years old). The researcher Dan Buettner called those areas "blue zones" in his 2005 National Geographic article "The secrets of a long life."[23]

There are common features among these elderly people from different areas of the world, which obviously contribute to a not only longer but also healthier life. One major component is their diet, which in all blue zone areas consists of a balanced, plant-based diet with whole grains, fava beans, legumes, and high polyphenol wine.

I was also involved years ago in the analysis of data from a cross-sectional study on occurrence of heart and vascular diseases on the Greek island of Crete, which formerly demonstrated one of the lowest incidences of heart problems in the world—until the people of Crete adopted a "Western diet" with fast food chains such as in the US (moving away from their traditional Mediterranean diet). As a result, within a few years, the former survival advantage vanished, and the Crete population developed similar levels of diabetes, high blood pressure, and heart disease as any other country in the Western world. In simple words, we are what we eat, and we should always stick to a healthy, balanced, plant-based diet rather than moving to processed food. Some people in age management medicine simplify the diet recommendations to their patient as follows: "If it runs, swims, flies, comes out of the ground, or falls off a tree, you can eat it."

Of note, several animal studies have now shown that a reduction in calorie intake does prolong life. Even though larger clinical human studies are lacking, I surely can attest that among more and more patients who are above ninety or even one hundred years of age who I see and examine on a weekly base, I have never seen an obese nonagenarian or centenarian.

Calorie reduction prolongs life.

The concept of a lower calorie intake has several supporters among age researchers, and there is also scientific data supporting the intermittent fasting concept (seventy-two hours of fasting can reduce oxygen-derived free radicals and strengthen the immune system).[24]

Another common factor among the centenarians in the blue zones is the lack of loneliness, meaning there is a social system that fully integrates older individuals into active participation within the community with the creation of a daily purpose for life.

Loneliness is a major factor in the Western world amongst middle-aged and elderly people, and it leads to depression, suicidal ideation, and early death. The existence of a social network without age distinction is ideal, in which the oldest and the youngest individuals can live together as a unit. This interaction enables the older people to stay youthful through the younger individuals, and the younger ones learn from the life experience of the elderly.

We have largely lost this close family and village connection as we are more focused on our core families or even single lives in our modern world, which does result in lack of communication and social engagement, particularly after the kids are out of the house and retirement from a regular daily work schedule. No wonder many people suddenly get sick once they retire after being healthy their entire working life. Having a purpose, a task, and a community is an essential aspect of a successful and satisfying aging process according to social study reports among the very oldest in the world.

Besides a balanced, plant-based diet and active social participation, there was another common factor amongst all these blue zones across the world. There was no exercise regimen among the elderly: no gyms, no workout routines, and no scheduled sport activities. This might seem surprising; however, a very active lifestyle without motorized transportation was still a common factor among the very elderly. In other words, even though they never saw a gym from the inside, they were physically active from a young age until the end of their lives by walking a lot within their community environments.

A healthy, balanced diet, physical activity, and a social network defy aging processes. Regenerative therapy can likely significantly support our natural response against degeneration with older age.

8.

In the News

Almost on a weekly basis, there are reports in the media, either in print, on TV, or on social media, about stem cell therapy and its success stories. I must emphasize that these reports are usually individual cases rather than large-scale, clinical trial data, but they foster the public's interest in regenerative medicine.

To give you an idea of the types of stories being widely shared, I list below several reports from articles in the *Daily Mail* from 2018 and 2019.

On **March 19, 2018**, a thirty-six-year-old female, Mrs. Louise Willetts, from Rotherham, UK, was featured as one of one hundred volunteers in a stem cell study to treat *multiple sclerosis* (a degenerative, incurable condition of the brain and the nervous system). The volunteers were either given conventional drug treatments or a "haematopoietic stem cell transplantation." The patients who received stem cells were treated with aggressive chemotherapy drugs prior to the stem cell transplantation. The stem cell transplantation involved using the patients' own blood to extract stem cells which were then injected back into the patients' blood. According to the online article, the stem cell treatment proved to be ten times more effective than drug treatment alone. The article also cited that three years after the study, an average of only 6 percent of patients treated with stem cells had a relapse of multiple sclerosis compared to the 60 percent of patients who received conventional drug treatments alone. The authors (and the patients) declared stem cell therapy might be a game changer for the management of multiple sclerosis, a chronic debilitating disease of the nervous system and the brain that cannot be cured and usually gets progressively worse.

On **April 4, 2018**, the *Daily Mail* reported that researchers from Columbia, New York developed a mature human heart muscle in a lab that will be useful in medical research dedicated to understanding more about heart disease and its possible treatments. Dr. Vunjak-Novakovic, a professor of medicine at Columbia University, and his team grew a mature human heart muscle from stem cells in four weeks by manipulating early-stage stem cells to accelerate the speed at which the cells developed into a mature human heart.

On **May 2, 2018**, it was reported that Prof. Nicholas Rivron of Maastricht University led a research team that successfully used stem cells to grow a mouse embryo without sperm or egg cells for medical research on infertility.

On **July 16, 2018**, the *Daily Mail* reported a story on Mrs. Pat Wilkinson, an eighty-year-old female from Winchcombe in Gloucestershire, who participated in a stem cell trial through the Compassionate Treatment Program by The Heart Cells Foundation. In 2016, Wilkinson received the stem cell treatment to treat her heart damage and cardiovascular system. The procedure was said to involve reinjecting her own stem cells directly into a vein in her groin from where the cells traveled to damaged tissue and encouraged new vessel growth and tissue regeneration. Wilkinson was given injections daily for one week. Wilkinson claimed to notice clear improvements within three weeks of the treatment, feeling "more energetic when climbing stairs" and enjoying walks without shortness of breath.

On **September 22, 2018**, a Welsh biotech company (ReNeuron) reported that more than half of the thirty-four patients who suffered from a stroke noted improvements in their condition after receiving stem cell treatments. The treatment involved growing neural stem cells in a lab using tissue samples from a US stem cell bank. Twenty million neural stem cells were injected into each patient's healthy brain tissue in a region close to the areas damaged during a stroke. This method was intended to release chemicals that stimulated growth of new nerve cells and blood vessels in the patient. According the ReNeuron's CEO, Olav Hellebo, a Manchester bricklayer who suffered from a debilitating stroke was eventually able to return to work because of the stem cell treatment he received.

Also, on **September 22, 2018**, the *Daily Mail* reported on Ms. Jodi Jackson, a forty-two-year-old female who received a stem cell treatment at the London Bridge Hospital (HCA Healthcare UK) for multiple sclerosis. This involved having her own stem cells extracted from her blood and bone marrow before receiving chemotherapy over a six-day period. Her cells were then transplanted back into her blood. Jackson said she suffered from hallucinations, nausea, burning pain, and mouth ulcers throughout the treatment and she was kept in a sealed room with purified oxygen. Five months after her treatment, Jackson said she was able to return to the gym four days per week and has the confidence to run the New York City Marathon. According to the follow-up reports, Jackson's latest MRI shows no active disease.

On **September 22, 2018,** the paper reported that Moorfields Eye Hospital and University College London treated two patients with age-related macular degeneration using embryonic stem cells that resulted in positive outcomes for both patients. Embryonic stem cells were converted into retinal cells in a lab through a process called spontaneous differentiation. The retinal cells that developed from the process were placed on a tiny membrane and injected just below the patients' retinas.

The two patients treated were an eighty-six-year-old male and a female in her sixties. Both patients' eyesight was so poor they were unable to read. The treatment resulted in improving the patients' vision enough to allow them to read sixty to eighty words per minute with reading glasses.

On **November 9, 2018,** the *Daily Mail* reported that researchers at the University College London were accused of covering up the deaths of two women that may have resulted from controversial stem cell procedures. Keziah Shorten, a twenty-year-old female from Kent, died following two separate treatments. The first was a stem cell engineered larynx transplant in 2010 to treat her failing windpipe. Shorten received another failed transplant in 2011 carried out by UCL and eventually died of pneumonia after six months in intensive care. Professor Paolo Macchiarini, who pioneered the treatment, was then an honorary professor at UCL and carried out Keziah's first transplant. Shauna Davidson, age fifteen from Teesside, died after a similar procedure in 2012. It has been reported that her transplanted trachea collapsed, suffocating her and causing fatal brain damage. She died thirteen days after the operation. The *Daily Mail* reports that the scientists deemed both operations successful and argued that Davidson died of non-graft related causes. Macchiarini was later found guilty of scientific misconduct by Sweden's Karolinska Institute because he failed to report the complications and deaths from his procedures in the research he published.

On **January 1, 2019,** the Cleveland Medical Center reported plans to conduct a clinical trial study in which twenty-four people would receive one of two doses of stem cells or placebo jabs to treat lower back pain. The researchers aimed to use stem cells to strengthen spinal discs by increasing water content to improve the cushioning between vertebrae, ultimately reducing inflammation and pain in the patients. The procedure would involve using stem cells from the patients' own bone marrow extracted from the patients' hip with a syringe. The stem cells recovered from the extraction would then be injected into the patients' spine. Results of this study were not published.

The *Daily Mail* reported on **February 4, 2019** that scientists were using stem cells to help find a cure for type 1 diabetes by replacing healthy beta cells destroyed in those suffering from the disease. Dr. Gopika Nair and his team of researchers transplanted lab-grown, insulin-producing cells that look and act like pancreatic beta cells into mice. The cells successfully produced insulin and responded to blood sugar within days of being implanted into mice. The findings have been published in *Nature Cell Biology* with hopes to find a cure for type 1 diabetes.

On **April 13, 2019**, the *Daily Mail* reported that tests on three American patients—two men and a woman—who were legally blind produced "exciting" results, according to Olav Hellebo, chief executive of UK biotech firm ReNeuron. It was stated that the three Americans' vision improved from being able to read only the largest group of letters on a special eye test chart to reading letters three sizes smaller on the same chart after the procedure. The treatment involves growing billions of progenitor stem cells in a laboratory. Approximately one million stem cells were injected into the back of each patient's eyeball where they would transform into new rods and cones replacing those that were lost prematurely to a genetic disease. One patient claimed that she is no longer classified as being "legally blind" after having the treatment. ReNeuron representatives reported that another patient's vision improved from being able to see just nine letters on the eye test chart to seeing twenty-nine letters.

The *Daily Mail* reported on **May 30, 2019** that Oscar Saxelby-Lee, a five-year-old male child at Birmingham Children's Hospital, received a stem cell transplant to treat aggressive leukemia. Oscar was diagnosed with T-cell acute lymphoblastic leukemia in December 2018 and received chemotherapy treatment. Donor stem cells were injected into Oscar's body so that they would turn into red and white blood cells to replace the patient's own cells destroyed by chemotherapy drugs. Replenishing the patient's blood cells would allow doctors to use higher doses of chemotherapy with less damage to his internal organs and immune system. The stem cell transplant would allow a more aggressive form of chemotherapy treatment to kill as many cancerous cells as possible without depleting the patient of vital cells.

Two female patients suffering from multiple sclerosis who had lost some control of their limbs due to the disease received autologous haematopoietic stem cell transplants as reported on **July 6, 2019**. Both patients said they received more traditional treatments to treat their multiple sclerosis symptoms prior to seeking stem cells as an alternative. Both patients have "… seen huge improvements since undergoing the procedure." One patient said that she suffered from pain feeling like pins and needles in her hands, as well as vision and coordination problems. The other patient reported improvements to the feeling of "tingling" in her spine and diminished leg mobility. One of the two women told *Daily Mail* that results from resent scans show no signs of active disease. The article reiterates that there is currently no cure for multiple sclerosis.

On **August 2, 2019**, the *Daily Mail* reported that research shows promise in treating heart failure using a combination of stem cells and heart cells to repair damaged tissue following a heart attack. Studies have been reported to show that stem cells helped heart muscles "grow again" and "improved their ability to contract and relax."

On **August 3, 2019,** a seventy-nine-year-old well-known American male actor reported receiving stem cell therapy treatments regularly to improve his appearance

On **August 10, 2019**, Chris Wild, a thirty-nine-year-old male from North London, was reported to have received a stem cell procedure that prevents and reverses hair loss. This specific procedure is associated with Ioannis Liakas of Vie Aesthetics in London with whom Wild received a consultation. The treatment involves having three small pieces of skin containing hairs and stem-cell rich fat taken from behind the patient's ear. Stem cells are extracted from the skin samples using a device called "Rigenera Activa," which is approved in the EU for extracting stem cells from hair, skin, and fat. Then, approximately 800,000 of the patient's own stem cells are injected back into the scalp, completing the thirty-minute procedure. Chris Wild says he sees improvement and new hair growth and that his mother noticed the same right away.

On **September 9, 2019**, the paper reported that Michael Schumacher, the famous Former F1 world champion who suffered severe brain injuries after a skiing accident would have injections of "secretome" (stem cell formula) into his veins that would result in anti-inflammatory effects that could possibly reach the brain. The article stated that Schumacher was under the care of Professor Dr. Philippe Menasche, who specializes in stem cell research and is known for stem cell procedures that involve grafting stem cells onto damaged tissue.

On **September 15, 2019**, the *Daily Mail* reported on James O'Brien, a forty-four-year-old man from London, who was blinded at eighteen years old in one eye as a result of having his eye sprayed with ammonia. He took part in an NHS eye surgery trial. The *Daily Mail* stated that stem cells were cultivated and grown in an Italian lab for six months using the man's own cells taken from his functioning eye. Surgeons at the Moorfields Eye Hospital used the lab-produced cells to replace the scar tissue from his blind eye. After one year, a cornea from a donor was inserted into the injured eye where the stem cells previously were said to ensure the cornea would function and restore his eyesight. The patient told *Daily Mail* that his eyesight has improved as a result of the procedure and the surgery has given him more confidence in himself overall.

There are tons more similar reports about anecdotal or studied stem cell therapies, and there appears to be a huge public interest in stem cell therapy in general.

9.

The Evidence

The safety and efficacy of adult stem cells have been intensively investigated for regenerative potential in clinical trials over the last twenty years. Due to the growing number of trials, it is becoming essential to cumulate and analyze the current status of those efforts. Therefore, my group aimed to extensively search and systematically review stem cell clinical trials. Since I am a cardiologist, I focus on cardiac and vascular diseases rather than other degenerative diseases or injuries.

In our review, we report the analysis of clinical trials using stem cells that are listed on the PubMed scientific publications database as of April 1, 2019, with an emphasis on their use in patients who suffered from a heart attack. Many ongoing registered studies were also included in this review. They can be viewed with a search on a clinical trial database, such as the NIH database (www.clinicaltrials.gov) and the European Union Clinical Trials Registry (www.clinicaltrialsregister.eu).

9.1 Heart/Vascular Problems and Stem Cell Therapy

What follows is an overview of heart and vascular diseases and the potential of stem cell therapy based on published data. The presented studies are but a brief summary of selected studies and the summary does not intend to be a complete review of all published data.

First, a heart attack or myocardial infarction is damage of heart muscle cells (necrosis) resulting from an acute obstruction (blockage) of a blood vessel of the heart (coronary artery). Heart attacks are still a major cause of mortality and morbidity worldwide and account for significant healthcare costs. In the US, approximately one million people suffer from a heart attack per year, and approximately 300,000 to 400,000 people die as a result of a heart attack per year in the US alone. Worldwide, more than seven million people have heart attacks per year.

The outcome of heart attacks has improved since the first percutaneous transluminal coronary angioplasty was introduced by the German physician Dr. Andreas Gruentzig in 1977. When Gruentzig approached his boss at the University of Zurich in Switzerland with the idea of placing a catheter into the artery of a patient with chest pain or a heart attack, he was thrown out with the words: "We are physicians, not magicians." Gruentzig then left conservative Switzerland and went to Emory University in Atlanta, GA in the US and quickly became the most prominent heart doctor in the world.[25] Gruentzig's success remains a major breakthrough and a great contribution to the field of medicine in demonstrating that doctors can work inside of the arteries safely without needing to perform open-heart surgery. Unfortunately, in 1985, he and his wife died in a plane crash when he was piloting.

Besides opening blocked arteries with catheter-based techniques, there have been significant advances in adjunctive pharmacotherapy, procedural techniques, and stent technology for the treatment of patients with heart attacks. However, the incidence, mortality, and morbidity due to heart attacks continue to remain high despite all these recent advances. Current in-hospital and one-year mortality are in the range of 5 to 6 percent and 7 to 18 percent, respectively.

Part of the reason for the high mortality rates is that heart muscle cells in adults have limited capacity for proliferating and self-healing. Once irreversible myocardial cell death has occurred due to ischemia, scarring inevitably forms, leading to adverse remodeling, reduction in left ventricular function, and subsequent heart failure or other serious adverse events, such as arrhythmias, and ultimately death.

Nowadays, with the development of regenerative therapy, stem cell therapy has become an attractive concept for heart repair and the restoration of cardiomyocytes and damaged myocardial tissue. More and more studies have emerged that explore the safety and therapeutic potential of stem cells in the context of ischemic coronary artery disease. Pluripotent stem cells possess the capacity to differentiate into all cell types of an organism, including mesodermal derived heart muscle cells (cardiomyocytes). However, in cardiac regenerative medicine, the therapeutic use of pluripotent stem cells is limited mainly due to the risk of immune rejection, genetic instability, tumorigenic potential, low efficiency, and ethical issues (for embryonic stem cells).

In past years, most clinical trials have tested autologous bone marrow derived stem cells because they are self-renewable and can be administered without adding any immunosuppressive therapy. Despite most experimental and clinical studies using bone marrow derived stem cells, these cells have limitations for clinical application, including an invasive harvesting procedure and decreased proliferation and differentiation, potentially related to donor age and comorbidity.

In contrast, umbilical cord derived stem cells are easily attainable and expanded in vitro, have less cellular aging, and are devoid of ethical concerns. Both human umbilical cord stroma and Wharton's Jelly can give rise to the isolation of clinical-grade cord blood derived stem cells used in allogenic cell injections to improve cardiac function. They possess immunomodulatory (enhancing the immune system), anti-apoptotic (protection against determined cell death), angiogenic (building new blood vessels), and anti-fibrotic (reducing development of scar tissue) properties.

In vivo experiments showed that umbilical cord derived stem cells could repair ischemic tissue by promoting the development of new blood vessels by means of neovascularization (the creation of new blood channels) and by reendothelialization (the repair of blood vessel cellular lining). Although the exact mechanism of action is still under investigation, the cells secrete certain factors and then transform themselves (transdifferentiate) into vascular cells to promote tissue regeneration.[26]

The immunosuppressive and anti-inflammatory properties of cultured and expanded umbilical cord derived stem cells have led these cells being tested for their therapeutic potential in preclinical animal models since the mid-2000s, and their differentiation characteristics and responses to the external environment have been extensively documented in vitro single and co-culture setups.

These are just a few of the major preclinical and clinical findings from the last several years. Preclinical studies have demonstrated that umbilical cord derived stem cells can express cardiac-specific molecules (troponin-I, connexin-43), differentiate into heart muscle and vascular cells in vitro, and exert paracrine effects that enhance vascular regeneration and cardiomyocyte protection.[27]

To date, three trials using umbilical derived stem cells to treat patients with acute heart attacks have been reported as full articles and another three ongoing trials are currently registered and underway. Also, one trial using umbilical derived stem cells to treat chronic coronary occlusion has been reported.[28]

Safety was targeted as the primary endpoint in almost all of these studies. Every author reported no adverse effects different between the treatment and control groups. In general, transplanted cells, ranging from three to 106 cells per patient, were found safe with no major adverse effects during and/or after the delivery of cells into coronary arteries via percutaneous coronary intervention.

As the secondary endpoint, the efficacy and feasibility of injected umbilical derived stem cells were tested in various delivery routes, such as direct injection into the arteries of the heart, into the heart muscle, or into the pericardial space (among other routes).

- Gao et al. conducted a randomized, double-blind, placebo-controlled study in 116 patients with acute heart attacks. After eighteen months of follow-up, the group reported a 7.8 percent improvement of cardiac strength measured by ejection fraction in the treatment group compared to 2.8 percent in the placebo-controlled group. Concomitantly, the absolute increase in the myocardial viability and perfusion with the infarcted territory was significantly greater in the treatment group compared to the placebo group. Significant improvements were also noted in the dimensions of the hearts at eighteen months. Adverse event rates and laboratory tests were no different between the two groups.[29]

- Musialek et al. applied umbilical derived stem cells to the coronary arteries in ten patients with first, large heart attacks and monitored them for twelve months for the safety of the procedure. They reported no adverse effects or significant arrhythmias; no data was given regarding the efficacy of the infused cells.[30]

- There is one study to investigate the safety and feasibility of intracoronary injection of umbilical derived stem cells to very old patients (aged eighty-one to ninety-two) with coronary chronic total occlusion conducted by Li et al. Fifteen patients received treatment. A 15 percent increase in cardiac strength after twenty-four months with a 21 percent decrease in infarct size area was found. Furthermore, an improvement of their functional capacity was reported. No cases of major cardiac adverse events were reported.[31]

Conclusively, umbilical cord derived stem cells were found safe and efficient in restoring cardiac function in a relatively short period after a heart attack in the studied patient populations.

However, there are certain discrepancies regarding the route of cell delivery, patient inclusion criteria, age range, state of disease, and duration of follow-up, all of which give rise to two main concerns in the efficacy of the therapeutic intervention: inconsistency of results and difficulty of cohort analysis due to the aforementioned variables. Therefore, for the clarity of efficacy, we suggest that precise inclusion and exclusion criteria should be considered for future studies.

9.2 Sexual Problems and Stem Cell Therapies

The prevalence of erectile dysfunction has increased in recent decades. Although many treatments offer some benefit for men with sexual dysfunction, unmet therapeutic needs remain, and promising new approaches are under investigation. One of these approaches is the use of stem cell therapy. We comprehensively reviewed published literature and ongoing phase 1 and phase 2 trials, and we identified twenty-seven trials using stem cell therapy to treat male erectile dysfunction. For details, please see our published review article on that subject in the reference list.[32]

Of the twenty-seven trials, three have been withdrawn, nine have published results, six are complete but without published results, and nine trials are ongoing or with an "unknown" status.

Erectile dysfunction is defined as the inability to achieve and/or maintain a penile erection sufficient to take part in satisfactory sexual intercourse. Erectile dysfunction is a common, major sexual disorder among men and can significantly impact quality of life for both patients and their partners. The Massachusetts Male Aging study (1987 to 1997) was the first large, community-based, random sample observational survey to study erectile dysfunction and showed that the condition was present in 52 percent of men age forty to seventy. The study also suggested that over 600,000 new cases of erectile dysfunction are expected annually in the US. Erectile dysfunction increases with hypertension, diabetes, heart disease, age, and lower education. Smoking, obesity, depression, psychological causes, and spinal injuries are also risk factors for developing the disease.

The American Urological Association guidelines suggest patients with erectile dysfunction see a mental health professional as adjunctive therapy, which has been shown to improve adherence to treatment plans and enhance the effects of other treatment approaches, resulting in improved erectile function. Other therapeutic options include noninvasive approaches, such as lifestyle changes or oral medications, in addition to more invasive treatments such as vacuum constriction devices, intraurethral and intracorporeal injection, and surgically implanted penile prostheses.

Most international clinical guidelines suggest the use of oral phosphodiesterase type 5 inhibitors (medications such as sildenafil and Viagra*) as first-line therapy because of their excellent efficacy and safety profiles. But these drugs do not work for everyone. Thus, unmet needs in treatment for erectile dysfunction have prompted the development of novel, minimally invasive therapeutic modalities, such as low-intensity shock wave and stem cell therapy.

In animal models of erectile dysfunction, the injection of stem cell derived secretomes restored the function of vascular cells in the penis, thus improving erectile function.[33]

- Bochinski et al. first reported in 2004 the injection of stem cells into animal erectile dysfunction models with penile nerve injury. Subsequent studies investigated the effects of stem cells treatment for erectile dysfunction caused by aging, diabetes, hyperlipidemia, and other etiologies.[34]

- In 2017, Hou et al. performed a meta-analysis of twenty studies that used a total of 248 animals with erectile dysfunction. The results showed that stem cell therapy dramatically increased the level of certain enzymes like neuronal nitric oxide synthase and cyclic guanosine that are responsible for the dilatation of penile blood vessels. Studies also showed that administration of a large number of stem cells led to a significant improvement in erectile function in diabetic animals.[35]

Because of these promising results in experimental animal studies, clinical translation of stem cell therapy for erectile dysfunction in men has emerged in recent years. This includes many phase 1 and phase 2 trials investigating the efficacy and safety of using intra-penile stem cell injections to treat erectile dysfunction.

We systematically reviewed literature on the clinical use of stem cells for erectile dysfunction, and we identified and screened 339 articles. Of them, nine articles reporting eight trials were found. There were 129 articles that were preclinical studies, 127 articles that were review articles, comments, editorials, and letters, and 74 articles were found to be irrelevant.

Safety is the primary endpoint for most studies (eight out of nine), and common sites of stem cell origin were adipose tissue, umbilical cord, placenta, or bone marrow. The injection was reported to be safe without major adverse effects during and/or after treatment.

The secondary endpoint was the efficacy of stem cell therapy, measured after a single injection or two consecutive intravenous injections.

All studies found a significant improvement in erectile dysfunction, as measured by established erectile dysfunction questionnaires, blood flow patterns in the penis, ultrasound measurements, and other parameters.

- In 2010, Bahk and his team reported the results of a single infusion of allogenic human umbilical cord blood stem cells in seven diabetic patients with erectile dysfunction who could not achieve an erection for at least six months despite medications. Following injection, blood flow into the penis, libido, and blood glucose improved without immune suppression. Similarly, all but one patient regained erections by the third month and maintained the ability to achieve erection over six months. The placebo-injected group experienced no changes. There were no safety concerns or adverse events during follow-up.[36]
- Another phase 1 trial tested the efficacy and safety of placental matrix derived stem cells in eight patients with erectile dysfunction. After the injection, three patients achieved erections without the help of any medication. Overall, this study showed that the treatment was safe, may enhance penile blood flow, and may improve erectile function.[37]
- Yiou et al. conducted a phase 1 and phase 2 clinical trial to treat post-radical prostatectomy induced erectile dysfunction using bone marrow derived stem cells. In twelve patients' refractory to maximal medical treatment, no serious side effects occurred. The authors found significant improvement of intercourse satisfaction and erectile function as measured by erection hardness scale and established questionnaires. At higher doses, they also reported a dramatic improvement in spontaneous erections. Improvements were sustained at one-year follow-up. In phase 2, six additional patients were included, no serious side effects occurred, and erectile function improved. Based on long-term follow-up data, the authors discussed that repeated injections might be necessary to prevent a gradual decline in erectile function over time.[38]

- In 2018, Haahr et al. revealed the results of a phase 1 clinical trial that included twenty-one patients with erectile dysfunction. All patients received a single intracavernous injection of autologous adipose derived stem cells freshly isolated after liposuction and were followed for one year. Eight reversible minor events were reported because of the liposuction and one patient complained of a scrotal and penile hematoma. These events resolved spontaneously at six months. Eight of the fifteen patients in the continent group had recovery of erectile function and regained the ability to perform sexual intercourse. The results again showed stem cell therapy to be well-tolerated and safe.[39]

- Recently, Demour et al. conducted an open-label, phase 1 clinical trial. Two consecutive intracavernous autologous bone marrow derived stem cell injections were given at baseline and thirty days later to treat four diabetic patients with refractory erectile dysfunction. Tolerability and safety were assessed immediately, twenty-four hours after treatment, and two years later. Efficacy was assessed at twelve months. The authors found significant improvement of erectile function scores, sexual desire, intercourse satisfaction, erectile function, and overall satisfaction.[40]

- In 2019, Protogerou et al. conducted a phase 1 study testing the safety and efficacy of treatment with adipose derived stem cells for patients with erectile dysfunction. Three-month follow-up revealed no severe adverse reactions during or after treatment except minor pain at the injection site, which resolved spontaneously. All participants reported increased morning erections.[41]

Since many patients do not respond to traditional therapies for erectile dysfunction, such as medications, intraurethral suppositories, vacuum-assisted erection devices, and others, it has become necessary to develop novel effective strategies to treat male erectile dysfunction.

When performing a Google search on the terms "erectile dysfunction" and "stem cells," 1,520,000 results appear within forty-eight seconds. Interestingly, the majority of these results represent advertising from venders trying to sell unapproved and undifferentiated stem cell therapies (for the treatment of sexual dysfunction). This social medial content stands in large contrast to the actual outcome of published data in the scientific literature. Despite a huge public interest in sexual dysfunction and stem cell treatments, only a few patient-data, proven, controlled studies have been published.

To date, there are nine published human trials using stem cell therapy for erectile dysfunction. Collectively, the results show significant improvements in penile hemodynamics and patients report improved erectile function scores. No major adverse effects were noted in these studies, and stem cell therapy has shown efficacy in erectile dysfunction resulting from many etiologies.

Most of the published studies (eight trials out of nine) followed patients for at least six months. Three published trials assessed efficacy at a twelve-month follow-up. Two studies reported sustained effect of treatment at one year, and the one with an even longer follow-up period (mean follow-up of sixty-two months) suggested a subsequent decline in the erectile function scores at one year after injection. Thus, it is largely unknown how long the stem cell treatment effect will last.

Published studies used a variety of stem cells derived from multiple sources. The cells were prepared using various protocols and administered at various doses, which might differentially affect treatment outcome. The specific mechanisms underlying stem cell efficacy in erectile dysfunction treatment have not been evaluated in clinical studies. Preclinical studies have shown that the differentiation of stem cells is not always present during the repair process and the therapeutic effects can persist regardless of cell numbers or even after the disappearance of the cells.

A current movement in the stem cell research community advocates a name change for stem cells to "medicinal signaling cells," which may reflect the broad effects more accurately. The cells secretomes hold several advantages over traditional cell-based therapies for regenerative urology. First, controversial issues associated with cell-based therapy, such as tumorigenicity, immunoreactivity, and mal-differentiation, might be circumvented by acellular secretomes. Second, secretome therapy might lead to development of over-the-counter treatments that are both more efficient and much cheaper than the cell-based therapy, which involves maintenance and expansion of individualized clonal cell populations. Finally, as the secretome is further characterized, its active components may be targets of molecular modification and tailored to the disease process of interest.

Of note, there are several studies that have not been published. In particular, there is one large-scale clinical trial enrolling more than a thousand patients over a ten-year period. We believe this listing has been initiated by a stem cell manufacturing company to sell products to potential physician clients and to encourage non-FDA-approved procedures. Using allogenic stem cells for the management of erectile dysfunction or any other condition is still considered experimental and is not FDA-approved.

Our own clinical allogenic stem cell study using umbilical cord derived stem cell secretomes is finalized and showing promising results, and the manuscript is accepted for publication in 2021.[42]

Despite several promising clinical results, a lack of high-quality evidence remains as most trials were not performed using a placebo group. Because less than one hundred patients have been reported to receive stem cell injections so far, future large-scale clinical trials with controls are necessary to assess the safety and efficacy of stem cell therapy for men with erectile dysfunction.

10.

COVID-19 and
Stem Cell Therapy

The COVID-19 pandemic changed our world in every single sense of the word. Who would have thought that a tiny virus found in a Chinese city most of us had never heard about before would suddenly overrun the world in its entirety, causing disease, death, social isolation, economic collapse, depression, job losses, and much more?

My team and I have been on the forefront of the treatment of COVID-19 patients during the pandemic. Its worst peak so far went from mid-December 2020 to mid-January 2021 with a person dying from COVID-19 every six to ten minutes in Los Angeles during that time.

While there is no curative therapy available, we learned a lot about how to deal with the disease in a year's time—using antiviral, anti-inflammatory medications, blood thinners, and respiratory therapy—but the outcome has been poor.[43] Now we finally have the vaccines on hand, at least in a step-by-step approach for healthcare providers and those at higher risk of dying from the virus such as the elderly and those with underlying high-risk factors like lung and heart diseases, frailty, diabetes, obesity, and dementia. Our group wrote a review article on current COVID-19 treatment options that is under review, as well as a hand booklet for the pandemic recovery which we finally may have reached.

Stem cells have been used to try to treat COVID-19 infections by our group as well as others; however, not much has been published so far. Initial data did come from Wuhan, China, where a Chinese doctor treated nine patients with a single intravenous injection of stem cells that, according to his statements, led to complete recovery of all patients. The data was presented in the *Daily Mail* but has not been published in any scientific journal as far as we know.

In addition, colleagues of mine who work at Cedars-Sinai Medical Center in Los Angeles published a six-patient case series on COVID-19 patients receiving cardiac derived stem cells with recovery.[44] A group from Miami also published a small, placebo-controlled study using stem cell injection with improvements in outcomes compared to placebo-treated patients.[45]

Our group did perform the very first placebo-controlled, randomized pilot phase study using umbilical cord derived stem cell secretome injections versus placebo in critically ill COVID-19 patients, and it showed a significant reduction in mortality in a small group of patients. The manuscript is currently under review for publication.[46]

Altogether, it makes absolute sense to consider using stem cells in the experimental setting for the treatment of an inflammatory deadly disease for which no cure is yet available. These initial promising results are likely caused by the anti-inflammatory response, in addition to possible reparative mechanisms in the lungs and hearts of affected patients and improved tissue perfusion and oxygenation secondary to possible angiogenetic effects, but this remains hypothetical until proven at large scales.

11.

The Clues to Anti-Aging: Adaptability

The ultimate question of scientists, philosophers, religious people, and most everyone at one time or another is: How long do we live—and how do we live? Can we do something to delay or even prevent the processes of aging? Can mankind gain the ultimate immortality?

All beings are made of cosmic energy, and energy never dissipates; therefore, in a way, there is immortality of energy. But that does not mean we can prevent diseases of aging and degeneration of our vital organ functions—so far.

If we think it through, evolution has taught us that immortality is possible to a certain extent. There are species that are immortal, such as certain bacteria and fungi that live almost forever and have learned to withstand extreme conditions such as extreme heat, cold, mechanical, or chemical aggression. They have learned to survive, and they are still alive. The term "biological immortality" is defined as a state in which the mortality rate from old age (senescence) is decreasing. Immortal species could still die from other causes, such as injuries. There is a myriad of ongoing research on preventing, reversing, or slowing down aging in both the experimental setting and clinical scenarios.

Taking a step back, let us think about how cells and humans can survive in a philosophical rather than biological sense. Let us consider survival to be synonymous with success. How can we be successful—as individuals or as single cells in a tissue conglomeration? Tons of smart people have studied the common denominators of success and of survival, and despite that fact that there are so many different conditions and hypotheses, let me narrow it down to one single characteristic that makes humans successful, that makes our cells survive, and that gives us an explanation for why stem cells do what we believe they do best. That single characteristic feature is: ***adaptability.***

The dictionary defines adaptability as the ability of an entity or organism to alter itself or its responses to changed circumstances or environments.

In the business world, adaptability is the ability to learn from experience and improve the fitness of the learner as a competitor in the business world. What does that mean in the real world? And what does that have to do with stem cell research and treatment? Let us dive into this fascinating world in order to understand where modern science might lead us in a few decades. I will start with a few metaphoric—but real—situations to demonstrate the value of adaptability.

One example I came across recently when listening to a TED Talk was the comparison between Netflix and Blockbuster. Netflix, as we all know, started as a small company shipping video discs and tapes to homes for a fee but then learned that the new environment of online media enabled adaptation to fulfill the requirements of the customers. Now Netflix has become one of the biggest websites for on-demand streaming.

In contrast, Blockbuster was a huge company with stores in every large and even mid-sized city in the United States where people could go into a store to rent movies. You would go in, pick a movie from a shelf, pay, rent it for two weeks, and then return the movie by dropping it off in the store's mailbox. Blockbuster did not adapt to the changing environment of online demand but instead insisted on sticking to their antiquated concept of having the go to the stores.

While Netflix became one of the most successful companies in the US, Blockbuster had to close all of their thousands of stores and cease all of their operations on November 6, 2013. Blockbuster is practically nonexistent to date as a result of its failure to adapt to digital demands. There are several critics in the business world who state that this example oversimplifies crucial concepts. Blockbuster did try to adapt to the digital demands by developing a digital platform that, in fact, for a short period of time was more successful than Netflix, but they ran into trouble with high customer fees and further mismanagement before putting their concentration back on the retail stores. Whatever the multitude of causes are in this particular example, the fact is that Blockbuster did not adapt appropriately to a new demanding environment, failed, and became bankrupt.

In another example, let me tell you the story of a friend I'll call Carolina. Carolina is a lovely, intelligent, attractive woman who worked in a position somewhat below her intellectual capacity in the same academic center as me. Carolina and I became friends, and it became obvious to me that she had issues with her coworkers (mostly female) who had worked in the institutions for many years. While Carolina thought that her female coworkers and supervisors did not like her because she was good-looking and "stole their show," I tried to explain that it was an aggressive but mostly fair environment where everyone must prove themselves to gain respect from others. "Swim with the waves" and "Show them that you are a team player" were my words to her on a few occasions. I then lost some contact and heard that she was fired after a month or so. I did not hear the exact reasons, but I can guess.

I then got her a job in another facility where I work and, guess what, the same thing happened after less than a year. Carolina told me, "I can't work with this person; she is a b**** and she hates me because men like me ... and she doesn't know anything and she is incompetent ..." and so on. I again tried to convince her to play it cool, to show her flexibility and willingness to work with the team. I even told her, "Just play a role, get their trust, and then you can ask for more or switch within the company to another position."

Well, Carolina did not do any of that, and as far as I know, she never returned to work. It's bad when a woman who really had great potential, but no sense of flexibility or adaptability, not only lost two jobs within a year but also burned bridges (which you never should do in the business and professional world). The lack of adaptive behavior in her work environment continued ruining her career (and I would not be surprised if this behavior caused more harm for her in the future in similar situations).

Adaptability is the one and only requirement for survival in any situation, whether it is in business, in school, at college, in jail, in a relationship, or in a Petri dish. Adaptability makes bacteria immune to hostile host conditions so they can survive and reproduce even in the presence of antibiotics that are supposed to kill them. Bacteria can develop resistance to antibiotics, thus surviving the treatment attacks physicians endorse. The coronavirus creates adapted mutations, leading to variants that might be even more transmittable or might require adjusted or repeated vaccinations in the near future. This is adaptability.

So why does nature allow or even invite adaptability? Well, mainly because we are in a constant process of evolution and development, and there is never a status quo since all life is basically energy that never disappears.

Stem cells, of note, are the only cells known to have inert adaptability in their nature that enables them to work in different environments, to adjust to different conditions, and to differentiate into different cell types on demand. That is the reason why these cells survive and can do their job, and we have to learn how to use them accordingly to improve repair mechanisms, fight diseases, and delay aging processes.

12

The Regulators and the Regulations

Stem cell therapies, encompassing collection, purification, manipulation, characterization, and delivery of cells for therapeutic purposes, have existed since the first successful bone marrow transplantations in 1968. Every physician who is considering using stem cell products in their office for patients, whether or not it is in the frame of institutional review board (IRB) approved clinical studies, should be aware that stem cell therapy in its current form (with the exception of stem cell transplantation for certain cancer treatments) *is not FDA-approved.*

Stem cell therapy is currently not FDA-approved.

Every patient considering stem cell therapy should also be aware the stem cell therapy is not FDA-approved.

Any healthcare provider involved in stem cell research or stem cell use should be aware of the exact FDA guidelines and recommendations.

Therefore, I have listed these in the details below, as a reference. Please keep in mind that things change and are in constant flux. For updated guidelines and recommendations, please visit the FDA website.

12.1 The FDA and Its Role

The FDA promulgated a regulation on human cells, tissues, and cellular- and tissue-based products issuing an appropriate regulatory structure for the wide range of stem-cell-based products that may be developed to regenerate damaged tissues. The publications regulating the use of cell therapy products are codified within the Code of Federal Regulations in the following sections: IND regulations (21 CFR 312), biologics regulations (21 CFR 600), and cGMP (21 CFR 211).

In particular, US federal regulation on cellular therapy is divided into two sections of the Public Health Service Act, referred to as "361 products" and "351 products." Traditional blood and bone marrow progenitor cells, as well as other tissues for transplantation, fall into the 361 products definition. The FDA has established that as cells or tissues used for therapeutic purposes, and the regulation that pertains to processing 361 products is coded under the Good Tissue Practice (GTP).

The European Union (EU) regulation (1394/2007) on advanced therapy medicinal products (ATMP) was entered into force in all European Member States in December 2008. The regulation makes reference to and is in coherence with the 2004/23/EC directive on donation, procurement, and testing of human cells and tissues and with directive 2002/98/ EC on human blood and blood components. This means that any use of human cells has to be in compliance with the quality requirements therein described. Both EU and US regulations are also clear on requiring that cells have to be prepared according to the good manufacturing practice for medicinal products.

In reviewing the FDA statements and regulations, one has to keep in mind what the role of the FDA is. For consumers—all of us—the FDA has the task of informing the public about any updates to information about how to stay healthy and safe. For patients, the FDA's role is to provide a forum for information about treatments, including alternative therapies, drug and device approvals, and public discussions about medical news. For healthcare providers, including doctors, the FDA has to publish medical product safety, adverse effects, and newly observed problems. For the medical industry, the FDA provides guidance for registration, listing, and regulations. The FDA also initiates criminal investigations in medical fraud cases.

For the purpose of our analysis, it is important to understand that in 1902, the Biologics Control Act was introduced, which later developed into the FDA's Center for Biologics Evaluation and Research (CBER). This center works under the leadership of Peter Marks, MD, PhD on the safety and regulation of biological products such as living cells, blood products or tissues (including stem cells), and genetically engineered immune cells for cellular or gene therapy. In this context, the center is supposed to oversee and regulate the quality of manufacturing biological products but also ensure their safety for human use.

As a regulatory agency, the FDA also issues warnings for deviations from common or approved clinical practices. The FDA—in contrast to the state medical boards—does not have the authority to take a physician's license away but has the right and executive enforcement power to shut down clinics that perform potentially harmful procedures for patients.

The FDA can also grant approval for drugs/medicines of life-threatening or life-sustaining technologies (so-called class III technology such as pacemakers or defibrillators) after a lengthy and intensive review process called premarket approval (PMA). The FDA then reviews scientific evidence from clinical studies that are usually provided by the manufacturers of the drug or the device. Of note, only 1 percent of products submitted for FDA approval pass this testing review. FDA approval for any given drug or therapy means that the agency has decided that the benefits of a certain therapy or drug outweigh the potential risks.

Over-the-counter drugs are monitored by the FDA as well for possible risks but do not undergo a rigorous approval process. Additionally, vitamins and herbal products do not need to undergo FDA review, but the FDA watches whether manufactures make any claims that these products treat or cure any diseases.

So-called low-risk medical devices (such as the stethoscope that doctors use to listen to the heart) are considered class I and do not require FDA approval. In contrast, class II devices are defined as nonlife-sustaining or life-threatening and do not require FDA clearance, which is usually granted if the manufacturer can convince the FDA that the device is equivalent to products that have been previously cleared by the FDA. The loopholes for this class have been abused by the medical tech industry in many instances to get devices cleared and marketed without appropriate scientific and clinical evidence since the clearance process is much less intense and rigorous.

The FDA has been repeatedly criticized for its failure to apply similar standards, its slow and delayed administrative processes to allow patients to benefit from newer technologies, and its questionable relationships with the medical industry. As an example, in 2015, the FDA spent $1.1 billion on the regulatory oversight of prescription drugs with 29 percent of the money provided by the US government ($331.6 million) and the remaining funds ($796.1 million) provided by drug companies. This is important to know in order to understand how the FDA works.

Altogether, the FDA's role as part of the United States Department of Health and Human Services provides executive power to protect consumers from exposure to low-quality, unproven, and potentially harmful therapies. The majority of their funding comes from the medical and pharmaceutical industries.

12.2 FDA Publications for Stem Cell Therapies

By reviewing the press and literature, it is astonishing how many statements have been publicized by the FDA about stem cell therapies. As representative examples, I include several FDA news releases between 2017 and 2019 below.

August 28, 2017: FDA warns US Stem Cell Clinic of significant deviations.

In this statement, the FDA issued a warning letter to the Florida-based US Stem Cell Clinic called Sunrise and its Chief Scientific Officer Kristin Comella for marketing stem cell products without FDA approval and for significant deviations from current manufacturing practice requirements, including some that could impact the sterile environment of their products and put patients at risk. The FDA criticized the US Stem Cell Clinic for using adipose derived stem cells for intravenous or intraspinal injections in patients with Parkinson's disease and other neuro-degenerative conditions, even though the FDA had not approved any biological products manufactured by this company. The FDA's commissioner, Dr. Scott Gottlieb, stated, "Stem cell clinics that mislead vulnerable patients into believing they are being giving safe, effective treatments that are in full compliance with the law are dangerously exploiting consumers and putting their health at risk ... As the FDA takes new steps to advance an efficient, modern approach to the regulation of cell based regenerative medicine, at the same time we will be stepping up our enforcement actions against clinics that abuse the trust of patients and, more important, endanger their health with unsanitary conditions or by purporting to have treatments which may not have any benefit."

These warning letters request a response by the clinics with a correction notice of deviations to the treatment of cell-based products.

On the same day, *August 28, 2017, the FDA released another statement targeting StemImmune, Inc* in San Diego, which administered stem cell treatments at the California Stem Cell Treatment Center in Beverly Hills and Rancho Mirage. In fact, the FDA seized five vials of Vaccinia virus (usually used only for high-risk patients such as military members exposed to smallpox viruses) that were obviously used to create a stem cell product for cancer patients by intravenous injections or direct injections into tumors. This kind of "stem cell therapy," in particular for cancer patients, puts patients at high risk for infections or autoimmune responses. Furthermore, long-term effects in the underlying cancer are unknown.

Dr. Gottlieb stated in an FDA statement on the same day that "… when cells are taken from and given back to the same individual or when the cells or tissues do not undergo significant manufacturing, they are intended to perform the same basic functions, and are not combined with another drug and device, among other factors, their benefits and risk are well understood. In these circumstances, the products may not require premarket review under current law."

In an article titled "*FDA warns about stem cell therapies*" there are several risks stated based on reports of a patient who became blind after in injection into his eyes and another patient who received an intraspinal injection that resulted in a growth of a spinal tumor. The risks of unproven therapies are:

- administration site reactions
- the ability of cells to move from placement sites and change into inappropriate cell types or multiply

- the failure of cells to work as expected
- the growth of tumors

On *January 4, 2018, the FDA posted a warning letter to the American CryoStem Corporation of Monmouth Junction*, New Jersey for marketing adipose derived stem cells under the tradename "Atcell," which according to the FDA underwent more than minimal manipulation without FDA approval. As in the above cases, according to Dr. Peter Marks, the FDA's director of the Center for Biologics Evaluation and Research, there is evidence of unsafe handling of the products that increased the risk of contamination, which itself could result in life-threatening reactions and infections in patients treated with the product.

On *May 9, 2018, the FDA then filed permanent injunctions in Federal Court against the above-mentioned US Stem Cell Clinic of Sunrise*, Florida and Kristin Comella, in particular for not responding to the warning issued August 28, 2017. Furthermore, the FDA filed a similar request for injunction to the California Stem Cell Treatment Center, Inc., with locations in Rancho Mirage and Beverly Hills, and Dr. Elliot Lander and Dr. Mark Berman for marketing their stem cell products without FDA approval. In both cases, the FDA found significant deviations from current good manufacturing practice requirements, including the lack of appropriate written procedures to prevent microbiological contaminations.

On *December 20, 2018, the FDA send a warning letter to Genetech, Inc,* of San Diego and its president Edwin Pinos for marketing stem cell products without FDA approval and for significant deviations from current good tissue practice and current good manufacturing practice requirements using processed umbilical cord products that were distributed by the marketing company *Liveyon, LLC in Yorba Linda*, California. The FDA stated herein that the umbilical cord products are intended for allogenic use, i.e., use not in the same patient who donated the cord blood but in genetically different individual patients, which means that the products are regulated as both drug and biological products. This in turn does require an investigational new drug application before it may be used in humans. Moreover, both the FDA and the Centers for Disease Control and Prevention are in possession of reports on twelve patients who received the Genetech and Liveyon-distributed products and subsequently became ill with localized (joint) or systemic bloodstream infections, including Escherichia coli related to the contaminated suspensions, which has been extensively reported in the press all over the country.

I have personally dealt with the above companies. Even though I do not know the details about the FDA's inspections, I do know that Kristin Comella, the CEO of the Florida-based stem cell clinics, is a well-regarded scientist in the stem cell arena. She actually developed several of the methods for how to separate stem cells from tissues and blood, and she also trains physicians from all over the country in these techniques. However, Dr. Comella is not a physician, and she is not actively treating patients, as far as I know.

I also dealt with distributing companies and, as a potential consumer, I was faced with enormous and very convincing marketing efforts but also a significant lack of any clinical or basic pathophysiologic or biochemical knowledge to back up any claims that were made. I decided to stay away from these companies.

One of the most promising evolutions in the world of medicine and science is the premise of stem cell therapies. This category of treatment is also one of the most controversial, as legitimate research and advancements against disease are often difficult to discriminate from speculative promises from unapproved stem cell clinics. The FDA is creating an extensive framework to promote the expansion of regenerative medicine products and has released regulatory consideration documents to summarize their commitment to groundbreaking stem cell research. These strict regulations allow the FDA to protect patients and assert manufacturer obedience of the law while staying on the path of efficient development of innovative regenerative medicine products.

Two final guidance documents clarifying the FDA's stance on whether a cell- or tissue-based product would be subject to the FDA's premarket review were released in November 2017, and a guidance for expedited programs for regenerative medicine for serious conditions was released in February 2019. Guidance documents released in *November 2017* by CBER were used to clarify existing regulations for sponsors to determine the need for premarket authorization for their products and to accelerate the development and approval of safe and effective innovative regenerative medicine therapies.

Laws applicable to human cells, tissues, and cellular- and tissue-based products (HCT/Ps) are Sections 351 and 361 of the Public Health Service Act. Section 351 states that the FDA requires manufacturers to hold a license in order to distribute HCT/Ps in interstate commerce; confirms that a product is safe, pure, and potent; and maintains the FDA's ability to suspend or recall products. Section 361 authorizes the FDA to issue and enforce necessary regulations to prevent introduction, transmission, or spread of communicable diseases from foreign countries into the US or between states.

Products can either be regulated by both sections or only section 361. Products regulated under both generally involve significant manufacturing and require clinical trials to demonstrate safety and efficacy. Those solely regulated by 361 undergo minimal manufacturing and can be assumed to be safe and effective; premarket review and approval is not usually required. In order to be regulated by section 361 only, an HCT/Ps must meet all criteria outlined by 21 CFR Part 1271.10 (a):

1. Minimally manipulated
2. Intended for homologous use only

3. Not combined with another article (some exceptions)
4. Either
   i. Does not have a systemic effect and is not dependent upon the metabolic activity of living cells for its primary function; or
   ii. Has a systemic effect or is dependent upon the metabolic activity of living cells for its primary function and is for autologous, first- or second-degree blood relative or reproductive use.

There is also a same surgical procedure exception under 21 CFR 1271.15 (b) that allows the product exemption from requirements in 21 CFR Part 1271. The exception applies when an establishment:

1. Removes and implants the HCT/Ps into the same individual from whom they were removed (autologous use)
2. Implant the HCT/Ps within the same surgical procedure
3. The HCT/Ps remain "such HCT/Ps" (they are in their original form).

The first step for determining if a product needs premarket authorization is to see whether the product meets the definition of an HCT/P. The following step is to determine if the same surgical procedure exemption 21 CFR 1271.15 (b) applies. If it does not, then the four criteria in 21 CFR 1271.10 (a) must be applied to see if the product can be regulated solely by section 361. If it does not meet all four criteria or if both sections 351 and 361 apply, additional requirements must be met, including the need to conduct clinical investigations under an investigational new drug application and to submit a biologics license application for approval prior to marketing. To allow manufacturers time to submit an investigational new drug application if needed, the FDA may give a thirty-six-month period of enforcement discretion for products if there is low risk to public health. Products with routes of administration associated with a higher risk, such as intravenous injections, aerosol inhalations, intraocular injections, or central nervous injections, are prioritized for regulations.

The Expedited Programs for Regenerative Medicine Therapies for Serious Conditions Guidance for Industry released in **February 2019** detailing provisions in the 21st Century Cures Act that allowed possible accelerated approval pathways for stem cell treatments. Regenerative medicine therapies to treat, modify, reverse, or cure serious conditions are eligible for FDA's expedited program designations: fast-track designation, breakthrough therapy designation, or Regenerative Medicine Advanced Therapy (RMAT) Designation.

Fast-Track Designation. If a stem cell product is considered a new drug that is intended to treat a serious condition, for which nonclinical or clinical data demonstrates the potential to address an unmet medical need in patients with such condition, it can receive a fast-track designation. Advantages include actions to facilitate development and expedite review of product. It could also be eligible for priority review if supported by clinical data at the time of marketing application submission.

Breakthrough Therapy Designation. If a stem cell product is intended to treat a serious condition, for which preliminary clinical evidence indicates that the product may demonstrate substantial improvement over available therapies on one or more clinically significant endpoints, it may qualify for breakthrough designation. The level of evidence needed for this designation is higher than fast-track designation. An example given in the guidance was that in advanced forms of age-related macular degeneration, subretinal administration of retinal pigment epithelium cells is associated with substantial improvement in either visual acuity or visual fields, or a substantial reduction in the area of geographic atrophy, at one year post-administration. The preliminary clinical evidence of substantial improvement over available therapies could be derived from phase 1 or phase 2 trials.

RMAT Designation. Stem cell treatments can be considered RMATs if they intend to treat, modify, reverse, or cure a serious condition and preliminary clinical evidence indicates that the regenerative medicine treatment has the potential to address unmet medical needs for such condition. It is essential that the preliminary clinical evidence be generated using the product that the sponsor intends to use for clinical development.

Priority Review Designation. Any product that received fast-track, breakthrough therapy, or RMAT designation may be eligible for priority review if it treats a serious condition and, if approved, would provide a significant improvement in the safety or effectiveness of the treatment of the condition. A decision regarding priority review grant is made within sixty calendar days of marketing application receipt.

Accelerated Approval. This has been used primarily in settings in which the disease course is long and an extended period of time would be required to measure the intended clinical benefit of a drug.

As stated by the CBER in the guidance, they will work with sponsors and encourage flexibility in clinical trial design for regenerative medicine therapies being developed to address unmet medical needs in patients with serious conditions, including rare diseases. For cellular or tissue treatments intended to replace a tissue or organ, CBER sees that evaluation of the long-term performance before marker approval would be difficult. For those products, CBER may consider short-term accomplishments as clinically meaningful results. Despite the many regulations surrounding regenerative medicine, there are considerations for those therapies that treat serious conditions.

The FDA is enforcing their regulations to confirm compliance and patient protection. In *May 2018*, the FDA filed for permanent injunctions against two stem cell clinics that had regulation violations in 2017. Both the US Stem Cell Clinic LLC of Sunrise, Florida and the California Stem Cell Treatment Center Inc. failed to address their violations in warning letters concerning marketing stem cell products without FDA approval and without correcting their violations of current good manufacturing practice regulations. The US Stem Cell Clinic was processing adipose tissue into stromal vascular fractions and intravenously or directly injecting the unapproved product into spinal cords of various patients with pulmonary fibrosis, Parkinson's disease, amyotrophic lateral sclerosis (ALS), and others. The California Stem Cell Treatment Center was using the live version of Vaccinia virus vaccine to create an unapproved stem cell product for intravenous treatments for cancer or direct injection into cancer patients' tumors.

In *December 2018*, the FDA warned Genetech Inc. of San Diego, California for marketing its processed umbilical cord blood into unapproved human cellular products that were distributed by Liveyon LLC. Twelve patients who received such products subsequently became ill due to blood and infections caused by various bacteria, including Escherichia coli.

In *March 2019*, the FDA issued a warning letter to Cord for Life president, Syed Raheel, for failing to qualify for any exemption, failing to meet criteria for homologous use, and for failing to follow preventative procedures for microbiological contamination.

In *April 2019*, the FDA sent twenty warning letters to healthcare providers and manufacturers who were suspected to be producing or marketing unsanctioned stem cell treatments, and FDA commissioner Dr. Scott Gottlieb promised continued efforts to stop illegitimate stem cell clinics. These actions exemplify the FDA's commitment to safe and legitimate practices in the field of regenerative medicine.

The emergence of stem cell treatments brings much promise to the world of science and medicine. Despite the rise of unauthorized products and unregulated treatment centers, the concept of regenerative medicine holds great potential in treating serious diseases. The FDA's strict regulations ensure that genuine and well-intentioned investigators and establishments are doing the crucial basics to develop quality products that are effective and safe for patients. With expedited program developments and more collaboration with legitimate developers, the FDA will hopefully remain committed in making those stem cell products accessible in the future.

Please also keep in mind that the FDA did not approve stents to be used in arteries of the heart for many years, even though cardiologists from all over the world showed its benefits. Just a thought. There is always *more to come from the FDA on these and other issues*.

13.

The Few Cases of
Serious Side Effects

The following serious side effects have been publicized after stem cell therapies.

Seventy-seven-year-old Doris Tyler from Florida with macular degeneration received stem cell injections in both eyes in September 2017 at a clinic in Peachtree City, Georgia, which is affiliated with the Cell Surgical Network founded by Dr. Mark Berman. The patient became blind as a result of bilateral retinal detachments a month after the injections. Three other women who received intraocular injections at the Florida-based US Stem Cell Clinic also became blind as reported in a New England Journal of Medicine article on March 16, 2017. A *Washington Post* article from April 3, 2019 states the FDA is suing the US Stem Cell Clinic in federal court at Fort Lauderdale, Florida.

On the contrary, based on a publication in *STEM CELLS Translational Medicine,* sixteen patients with limbal stem cell deficiency with impaired sight were treated with allogenic corneal epithelial stem cell administration and nine out of sixteen patients had significant improvement in their vision (while no one in the control group had any improvements). This data was widely publicized on March 10, 2019.

On December 18, 2019, and several times thereafter, several media outlets, including the *Washington Post* and the *New York Times*, reported that twelve patients became seriously ill from infections caused by contaminated stem cell products manufactured by Genetech and distributed by Liveyon. All of these patients needed hospital admissions and treatment for twelve to fifty-eight days. Thankfully, the company responsible for the distribution of those cellular products shut down at the end of 2019, although they did open back up last I heard.

While there have been other side effects reported, the majority of press releases about stem cell therapy have been positive with regard to impressive functional improvements for many conditions. Our group published an analysis on stem cell studies done in patients with heart disease a few years ago which overall showed only minor side effects.[47]

14.

Talk to Your Physician

Whenever you or one of your family members consider a treatment or develop new symptoms like pain or functional impairment of an organ, you consult with your doctor. It's that easy. Your doctor will then advise you on a possible diagnosis (or at least a working hypothesis for what they believe is wrong with you) and then likely will order some tests to verify or rule out a diagnosis. They might also recommend some initial treatment using medications or procedures to improve your symptoms and prevent possible deterioration or irreversible damage. Your doctor then will ask you to follow up within a certain time period to be reevaluated and adjust the therapy plan (or stop if the initial problem is solved).

For example, if you consult your doctor because you are having pain when you urinate and you show increased frequency of urination (the symptoms), the doctor's working hypothesis (or suspected diagnosis) likely will be a urinary tract infection (UTI). You likely will then receive a prescription for an antibiotic for a week and a recommendation to stay hydrated with an increased daily liquid intake. The doctor then might also recommend a urine analysis to verify the diagnosis of a

UTI. You also might be asked to come back to the clinic after two weeks if symptoms persist.

This is an example of how the majority of doctors in the world would handle a standard case. Physicians' actions are generally universal and somewhat streamlined, since the study and the practice of medicine is more or less identical worldwide. This is the ideal and best-case scenario whenever you consult a doctor. You can expect an identical generalized professional evaluation whether you go to the primary care doctor around the corner from your house, an urgent care facility to talk to an emergency physician, or a professor in a major university hospital.

While that might be the case for painful symptoms of a urinary tract infection, it gets a bit more complicated for the management of chronic debilitating diseases such as multiple sclerosis or congestive heart failure. Therefore, more and more patients are seeking additional advice from specialists in particular areas, such as a neurologist for multiple sclerosis or a cardiologist for heart failure, or even another super specialized cardiologist who is board-certified in advanced heart failure and transplant cardiology. In most cases, a primary care doctor will initiate the referral to the specialist, and in some cases, the specialist will then refer the patient further to the super specialist. However, this process is not common standard even though it is used often.

Let us assume you are a patient with congestive chronic heart failure and you have seen your primary doctor or general practitioner, an internist, and then a cardiologist. You are on all the right medications, such as a beta blocker, an ACE inhibitor, an Aldosterone antagonist, and aspirin, but you feel lousy. You end up in a hospital every few months for worsening symptoms. Somehow, you just don't feel better, and you want to look into further treatment options.

In that case, many physicians might tell you that there is nothing else to do except adjust medication dosages. Very few doctors will refer you to a large academic center with expertise in advanced heart failure treatment like left ventricular device implants or heart transplantation. Let us assume now that you feel it is too early to consider such extreme and life-changing surgical treatments, but you've heard about stem cell therapy for heart failure in the media.

You then might ask your doctor(s) about that, and most likely everybody will tell you that is it not FDA-approved, it is not paid for by insurance companies, and there is not enough data to recommend a generalized adoption based on few anecdotal publicized reports in the media. And this would be the correct recommendation, in general.

While some physicians might even tell you not to think about nonapproved therapies, others might encourage you to look into it more closely.

Why is there a difference in what different physicians will recommend? Let me explain the pitfalls that the general public doesn't know from an insider view so you can understand why some physicians may be open to novel treatment approaches while others are completely against it.

In this chapter, I provide the following four lessons and explain them based on my personal experiences with colleagues over the last decades. In no way do I intend to discriminate doctors or patients—just the opposite. I will show you today's real world of medical care, which might be somewhat surprising, by giving you a few examples of my very personal experiences as a doctor who has been around doctors all my life.

The four lessons are as follows:

- Lesson 1: Doctors are humans
- Lesson 2: Doctors follow rules
  - Doctors try to help the patient with the best available medicine
  - Do not do any harm
  - Doctors need to protect themselves
- Lesson 3: Doctors have a business
- Lesson 4: Patients are humans

14.1 Lesson 1: Doctors are Humans

When I grew up, there was one doctor in the next village. I will call him Dr. S. This doctor was a very well-respected man; everyone knew him in the community. If he walked through the town on a Sunday, everyone greeted him by his title and name. He also was known as a very busy man, and he lived in a large house with a huge yard and many large white dogs (Great Pyrenees), and he drove a large but always dirty Mercedes. He frequently came to our house on the weekends since he adored my father's red wine collection (and drank a lot of it). Dr. S. was it; he was the only show in town, and everyone went to him, trusted him, and asked no questions.

Dr. S. was a general practitioner, and as far as I remember, he was a good physician and a nice human being.

Years later, when I was in residency in internal medicine fifty kilometers away from my hometown, I encountered different types of physicians. Among others, I came across Mr. H., a physician who never received a doctoral degree (which is possible in Germany since someone can be a physician without being a doctor). I was the newest—and completely inexperienced—first-year resident. I had just come out of medical school with a huge amount of theoretical knowledge in my head but zero clinical experience. I also had just finalized both of my theses and was awarded the doctor titles from both the Universities of Vienna and the Philipps University in Marburg (In many European countries, physicians cannot use the title of doctor unless they have done research and published a thesis and then they will be awarded the doctor title from their university, whereas in the US and most other countries physicians automatically are called doctor. Therefore, in Germany, a person can be and work as a physician, but he or she cannot put the Dr. or MD with their name unless they have earned that title).

Mr. H. was a senior physician without a doctor title, while my inexperienced self was a physician without a clue but with two doctor titles before my name (Dr. Dr. or MD, PhD). Naturally, Mr. H. did not like me from day one and made that very clear. He never talked to me directly and only in the third person, even in front of me (e.g., "Who does he think he is, that beginner?"). In addition to being a complete butthead toward a youngster who tried to learn from a more experienced colleague, it did not take long for me to realize that Mr. H. was a good talker when communicating with patients but, in reality, he was an unresponsive physician whose ignorance and laziness endangered patients' lives on several occasions. Worse, he abandoned patients and was finally terminated from his job in the hospital.

He then started working in a private practice setting, and I do remember an older lady living above my apartment in the middle of the city telling me that Mr. H. (whom she called Dr. H.) was such a great man and a wonderful doctor. I thought, "If you only knew about this guy's unethical, unprofessional, and dangerous behaviors." I did not however, share my personal experiences with Mr. H.

I could fill pages with the unethical behavioral patterns
I encountered with this colleague of mine, but again,
I am not here to speak poorly about any individual.
In any case, I thought that this practicing physician was
a bad one, and most of my former colleagues felt
the same and never sent patients to him.

Years later, on my first day at a large academic university hospital, I was walking late in the day toward an elevator, but I was not sure where I was in the huge, 1,000-bed facility that was very confusing to navigate for anyone new to the institution. I then spotted a little man jumping up and down in front of the elevator. He started kicking the elevator door with his cowboy boots and screaming at the door. I didn't dare come closer since I was afraid and thought that I might be somewhere in a closed psychiatry section with an escaped patient.

I went to the closest nursing station and called the security desk about that strange little man screaming at the door. Security came after a few minutes but left me embarrassed on my very first day. I had no idea how I found the courage to come back the next day (or stay at that institution for the next ten years).

It turned out that the little man was Professor Dr. M., the head and chairman of a surgery department, an absolute genius in the operating theatre with a worldwide indisputable reputation as a doctor and surgeon. Of course, he had a very extroverted mentality, the loudest voice when screaming one can imagine, exhibiting the classical "little man syndrome."

In my experience over the coming years, I learned that this man was a fantastic physician and a world-class surgeon, but his personality outside the operation theatre was very difficult to handle at times.

Years later, when I lived in the Middle East, I had an opportunity to work with a heart surgeon, Dr. I., who actually did absolutely nothing.

His practice was to strictly follow the Hippocrates oath: do no harm. In order not to do any harm, Dr. I. decided just to do nothing, to refuse patients, and to refuse any surgical procedure. Since he had a five-year contract, he just avoided any medical complications by doing absolutely nothing (which would be impossible in the US or in Western Europe).

I must assume that his decisions were the result of laziness and lack of any interest in any patient's fate, as well as the lack of need to do any work since he was paid just to be around as a heart surgeon. Maybe that was even a smart move on his part, although not compatible with my ethical standards.

In my opinion, and after I had many arguments about patients needing surgery with this individual (which they did not receive at that institution because of his refusal), Dr. I. refused to provide any medical service at the cost of patient care in order not to be bothered.

Later, when I worked in a large Los Angeles academic institution, I came across Dr. C., a senior physician who had been at the institution for decades. I must admit that I had never met a physician with such a dedication to truly helping people without any regards to limiting factors. Though obsessive compulsive and sometimes difficult to communicate with, Dr. C. hardly ever left the hospitals before 10 p.m. after early morning hours. He was a true fighter for any possible treatment for every single one of his patients. During his brief vacation periods, Dr. C. went on medical missions organized by his church in Africa, Asia, or Latin America to help sometimes hundreds of patients per day with basic medical needs.

In my opinion, Dr C. was, and is, a dedicated, hard-working, responsible physician and humanitarian—a role model for others.

These are just a few examples from a selected group of physicians I came across in my career. These examples should demonstrate just how different doctors can be. It is true. Doctors are humans, after all, with their strengths and their mistakes. Some are great human beings and fantastic doctors while others might not be at a level high enough for me to send any person close to me for treatment by them.

14.2 Lesson 2: Doctors Follow Rules

The study of medicine is relatively regulated and is more or less identical all over the world with the exception of local or traditional arts of medicine that are different across the globe. Most medical schools at universities have adapted the US curriculum. The USMLE (United States Medical Licensing Examinations) can be taken anywhere in the world in specialized learning centers. All physicians go through medical school attending courses in biology, physics, chemistry, biochemistry, pathology, pathophysiology, and anatomy. Besides a few new developments, the basics in subjects like chemistry or anatomy haven't changed much over the last century.

Practicing medicine nowadays is guarded by "evidence-based medicine" and somewhat dictated by standardized guidelines. These guidelines are published papers outlining the evidence of certain diagnostic procedures and treatments usually based on large-scale randomized clinical trial data as well as expert opinions. The guidelines mention different classes of evidence. For example, to implant a pacemaker in a patient with a very low pulse rate as a result of a complete electrical block in the heart (an electrical block rather than a blockage in a blood vessel) is a ***class I recommendation*** if the patient has symptoms such as passing out or severe dizziness and if the patient has a reasonable life expectancy and no major contraindications to the procedure. This level of evidence is based on clinical trial data that supports such a treatment. On the other hand, to implant a pacemaker in a patient who had a few episodes of low heart rates during the night without any symptoms and without a heart block would be a class III recommendation, meaning that this procedure would be unnecessary and potentially harmful for the patient.

These guidelines are published by the medical societies and experts in the fields. They are not rules, but they do represent what a reasonable doctor would and should do or not do in a particular case. While the practice of medicine has to be individualized to the needs of each particular patient, the guidelines serve as a frame in which doctors should practice medicine.

In case of a bad outcome, for example, a patient dying as a result of a non-recommended treatment (a class III recommendation), this would likely represent a deviation from standard practice guidelines and the doctor might be subject to penalty.

Lawyers for malpractice cases in medicine love guidelines, since it is relatively easy to assess whether or not a particular doctor followed these recommendations. While medicine in Europe adhered more freely during the last decades, US doctors must strictly follow guidelines in order to avoid being accused of doing something that might not be considered standard of care.

Practicing medicine nowadays is based on the following three principles:

1. Doctors try to help the patient with the best available medicine
2. Do not do any harm
3. Doctors need to protect themselves

Try to help patients with the best available medicine

This in itself should be a no-brainer, and that is what doctors usually do. We evaluate patients based on their symptoms, their history, and their risks, and then we recommend diagnostic tests and therapy, whether those are medications or procedures. Whatever a doctor recommends, however, is a suggestion based on his expertise and current guidelines. It is the doctor's job to explain why they recommend a certain treatment, the possible side effects, and alternatives. All this must be documented in the patient's electronic medical record. Most patients then might decide to follow the doctor's recommendations, while others might not. If the patient suffers from pain, for example, they likely will follow the recommendations. If the patient does not feel anything bad, such as is the case with high blood pressure, they might not want to take medicines proven to prevent long-term damage. No one can be forced or talked into any therapy or procedure (even if it may be lifesaving) since, in the end, it is always the patient's decision whether or not to follow the doctor's recommendations. The doctor's job is to explain and advise, and if agreed upon, to initiate the appropriate most advantageous and least harmful diagnostic and therapeutic steps.

Do not do any harm

Any treatment, any drug, any pills, any procedure can have side effects. If a doctor tells you there are no side effects, run. It is our obligation to mention side effects and risks to every patient, but that does not mean that every patient will develop these side effects. I have had several patients tell me that another doctor prescribed a certain blood pressure medication (amlodipine, a widely used calcium blocker used for the treatment of hypertension that usually is very well-tolerated), but in their individual cases, the drug caused severe leg swelling. As a result, many of these patients decided it was the doctor's fault, that he gave them the "wrong medication," and they never went back to see that doctor again.

Of course, the doctor should have told the patients that amlodipine, though a great medication to reduce and control high blood pressure, can have leg swelling as a possible side effect. Leg swelling occurs in less than 10 percent of patients taking amlodipine, meaning it does not occur in more than 90 percent of patients taking it. These facts and possible side effects need to be emphasized to patients, and that is the same for any drug therapy. There is no way for the physician to determine whether his patient will develop leg swelling. This has nothing to do with being a bad doctor or prescribing the wrong medication, even though some patients might feel that way.

We as physicians also know that several medications can do harm, such as some chemotherapeutic agents can cause heart failure. In such cases, risks versus benefits need to be discussed with the patient and a consensual decision between healthcare provider and patient should always be attempted. It is, at the end, a shared decision-making process for or against any treatment. If a patient decides against a particular treatment or against any treatment at all, then that is their right to do so as long as they understand the possible risk and consequences of no treatment.

Doctors need to protect themselves

Physicians needs to protect themselves against malpractice as well as wrongful allegations. This is usually done by adhering to practice guidelines, as outlined above. As long as physicians follow the standards of care, they protect themselves somewhat against allegations from patients, their caregivers, colleagues, or even from lawsuits.

In the US in particular, doctors are much more careful with regard to following guideline-directed management, whereas in other parts of the world, doctors sometimes have the ability to think more outside the box and might be more willing to try more experimental approaches in individual cases. If experimental medicine is practiced, however, it needs to be clearly stated to the patient, who usually has to sign an informed consent form saying they understand the experimental and nonapproved nature of the procedure.

This should be standard practice currently for most stem cell therapies. Some physicians think if they have a study protocol for an institutional review board that this alone makes the use of stem cells or other experimental therapies legitimate, but for legal reasons, that is not the case. Most physicians join larger groups or medical societies that can provide a framework for legal advice.

In general, physicians should stay away from performing unapproved treatments. In the case of the promising world of stem cell therapy, it is advised to contact the FDA, follow the recommendations, and get in touch with professional societies or groups who regularly deal with the legal aspects of nonapproved therapies.

14.3 Lesson 3: Doctors Have Businesses

The fact that being a physician is a business should not be underestimated. Whether a doctor is employed by a hospital, a university, a medical group, or is an independent single practitioner, at the end of the day, it is a business for the doctor to earn money and feed their family.

With several changes in reimbursement over the last decade, many doctors are looking into areas outside their expertise to make money. The public does not have a good grasp of the reimbursement reality of a doctor since doctors were considered high earners in the past. Even though doctors are usually making a good living, please be reminded that most doctors work very hard and do not have nine-to-five jobs. Many doctors are on call twenty-four-seven for their own patients every single day of the year and often have to perform emergency procedures in the middle of the night after fourteen hours of hard work during the day.

I was on STEMI (acute heart attack) calls for a while and usually had to rush to the cardiac catheterization laboratory in the middle of the night to save a patient's life by opening an acutely blocked heart blood vessel with balloons and stents. Of course, it is rewarding to save a person's life and the highest form of giving a helping hand for someone in need, but the reimbursement for such procedures that might last for several hours is very low, and if patients have no insurance, often no payment is provided whatsoever.

Medicine is a healing art and a highly sophisticated science, but medicine also is a business. Many nonmedical or pseudo-medical companies try to feed off this business by selling products or services to doctors, which can then lead to the usage of unapproved testing or therapies.

Doctors in general have to be careful not to adopt promised therapies because someone from the industry tries to sell them something that might increase their business revenue. I remember one time a group of local businesspeople came to me with a patient they brought in. This patient was from out of state and obviously found something about this company on their website that promoted some kind of immunotherapy to strengthen the patient's weak heart. The company claimed to use the patient's own blood to create an immune cocktail that was supposed to result in improvement of the heart's contractile strength.

Upon my questions about how the blood is treated after it was taken from the patient and what manipulation would be done before reinjecting the cocktail into the patient's bloodstream, I received some generalized claims that were neither published anywhere nor could they provide me with any scientific data or any regulatory license or FDA registration for their product and therapy.

They had already charged the patient several thousands of dollars and offered me a fee to inject their cocktail.

This particular patient had a double heart valve replacement many years earlier and was a high-risk case. The patient was also evaluated in an outside academic hospital facility and advised to be evaluated for heart transplantation. The patient did not want that; therefore, she and her family looked into other treatment options. The easiest way to find "alternative treatments" is—of course—via internet searches. In many cases this is just misleading since the majority of reports on such treatments are sponsored by companies to promote their products rather than based on any reliable scientific data.

Any injection of contaminated blood products could easily cause a life-threatening infection because of the risk of artificial heart valve infection (endocarditis). For that reason, among others, I advised the patient against this kind of treatment and refused to do the injection. In addition, there is no scientific evidence whatsoever to prove any concept of efficacy with regard to the company's claim that her heart function would improve, nor was any safety data provided.

The patient and her family were mad at me since they were hoping that I would help them in the way they were expecting based on false promises from nonmedical businesspeople who tried to make money off of someone's sufferings.

My take and my recommendation based on my assessment was to stay away from unapproved "treatments" and be evaluated for a heart transplant. The patient never came back to me. I would not be surprised if this company tried to recruit another doctor to give the injection to the patient, which I hope never happened, for the patient's sake.

There are black sheep among doctors, too. I don't suppose there are that many, but there are some who might prioritize business interests over their profession to promote and support health. In our society, however, the medical societies, the regulatory agencies, and the insurance companies keep a closer eye than ever on physicians. All the black sheep will get caught at some point, as always.

Earlier I mentioned one of my experiences visiting an anti-aging medical conferences where I was invited as a speaker. It was a relatively small conference with approximately 150 doctors attending. The attendees were mainly physicians who practiced geriatric medicine and/or some kind of alternative medicine in their offices. Only a year later, I was presenting again at the same conference, and, at that point, there were more than 600 attendees. These doctors came from all specialties, from primary care to plastic surgery to gynecology to orthopedics to sports medicine to cardiology. The fact that there is so much more interest in "anti-aging medicine" is based on several factors:

1. Doctors are looking for different ways to make an income, some by selling products in their offices and others by providing some form of anti-aging and preventive medicine. This is a business interest.

2. Patients are actively asking their doctors about supplements and other "alternative" ways to treat certain chronic conditions beyond the classical treatment approaches, i.e., there is a huge demand from the patient side.

3. Most practicing physicians in this country are now in the baby boomer age, i.e., they themselves have a personal interest in staying young and healthy.

14.4 Lesson 4: Patients are Humans

As doctors, we are supposed to treat every single patient with dignity and respect. I believe that the vast majority of physicians perform their duties accordingly. On the other hand, patients are humans too, and, as physicians, we all have encountered difficult patients. Difficult does not mean difficult in terms of a medical challenge like serious multi-morbidities. That's the kind of challenge most physicians like to deal with.

But we all have seen patients who are extremely demanding, oftentimes noncompliant with recommendations, and then complaining that they did not get any better. Noncompliance with medication recommendations is a major problem. For example, the number-one reason for hospital readmission for patients with chronic congestive heart failure is noncompliance with medications or fluid and salt restrictions. That means that patients don't take their water medications as prescribed and then end up with swelling in their legs and water in the lungs.

The reasons for noncompliance often include a lack of understanding and a lack of resources, i.e., patients run out of their medications and then cannot afford to buy them again. After the economic crisis in 2008, we actually performed a study that showed that the number of hospital admissions was significantly increased due to the fact that many people lost their insurance coverage.[48]

For all these reasons, it is important to stress education for patients and their caregivers about their condition and the need for medical therapies. This is a time-consuming process, and doctors often lack the appropriate time to explain detailed information.

We as doctors also have encountered patients demanding procedures or surgeries that are medically not indicated. I remember one patient who requested an open-heart surgery for an aortic dissection (a partial rupture of the main artery in the body). It turned out that he did not have an aortic dissection as per imaging findings, but the patient also stated that he had a heart transplantation done at the Medizinische Hochschule in Hannover, Germany many years ago, and he was on immunosuppressive medications usually prescribed after heart transplantation. Since the patient did not really need another open-heart surgery, he got angry at the treatment team of doctors, including myself, and requested to be operated on immediately because of severe chest pain.

Well, the treatment for chest pain is definitely not surgery, and when I told him that, he got even more angry. Something was odd about this patient. Since I know the heart transplant team in Hannover, Germany from my ten years working at the RWTH University, I called them up. When I asked about this patient, the very first response on the phone was: "Not again." It turned out that this patient never had a transplantation in Hannover, and every month that particular university hospital received calls from different hospitals all over the US to inquire about that particular patient.

Moreover, it turned out that he actually never had a heart transplant whatsoever, but he had a sternotomy scar, i.e., someone in the past obviously opened up his chest (likely for suspected aortic dissection) but nothing was done in the end since he did not need any surgical repairs. When I confronted that patient with these obvious facts, he ripped out his IV line and left the intensive care unit and the hospital screaming and yelling (against medical advice).

Approximately six months later, I received another call form the intensive care unit to consult on a patient with a prior heart transplant in Germany. This was the same guy, admitted under a different name, with a different social security number, and he again requested open-heart surgery for severe chest pain. When I saw the patient, he again ripped his IV lines out and ran out of the hospital. Interestingly, he was taking immunosuppressive medication to avoid rejection of the transplanted organ, even though he never had any transplant. This is an extreme example of Munchausen's syndrome, a psychiatric condition where someone has a pathologic fascination with a nonexistent disease for secondary gain such as attention or pain medication. What I learned from this and other examples is not to believe anything unless it is verifiable and documented.

This is an extreme case; however, it should remind us that patients are humans, too.

15

The Remaining Questions

n brief, many questions remain unanswered regarding the status of stem cell therapy. Despite all the published and ongoing studies and the fact that all published trials have shown at least some benefits of stem cell therapy, there is still no consensus on several issues, such as:

1. Which stem cell origin is the best option for the condition being treated?
2. How many cells need to be administered: five million, thirty million, one hundred million cells? How many do we need to show best results?
3. Which route of administration of cells is optimal? Intravenous? Direct injection in affected organs? A combination?
4. How long does the effect last? Is there a need for a booster after one month/one year/five years?
5. What is the best way to ensure the cells best potential/viability/probability to survive in the recipient's organism?
6. Is there a need for a mediator/stimulator/combination of trigger factors to activate the cells?

7. What measures of quality control are in place for the isolation/preparation and administration cells?

8. When—if ever—will stem cell therapy be approved by the FDA and when will the costs be covered by medical insurance companies?

I do not have good answers for any of the above questions. Only ongoing and further controlled, high-quality research efforts can help us shed more light on the unsolved issues before stem cell therapy can be considered a widely used therapeutic option for many of us and our patients.

16.

For Health and Beauty

Similar to anti-aging movements is the everlasting goal to look young and beautiful. There are tons of stem cell products people can buy for skin improvements. Those products usually contain plant-based stem cell products in creams or gels that when applied to the surface of facial skin or body skin might or might not have an effect on the underlying layers. However, our group has used stem cell injections extensively for facial rejuvenation purposes in men and women at middle and advanced ages. Stem cells clearly have the potential to repair skin damage, improve blood supply within the skin (which helps with regeneration and repair mechanisms), and promote cellular turnover and increase collagen production. In particular, increasing collagen production can result in a reduction of fine lines and wrinkles and improvement in skin texture, tone, and elasticity. As a result of stem cell injections in the skin, the facial appearance is usually younger and more vibrant. From our anecdotal experience over the last fifteen years, most of our patients come back in regular intervals (every six to twelve months) because everyone likes healthier, younger-looking skin. A combination of stem cell injections with certain plant-based stem cell products might create additional benefits for skin anti-aging purposes. These stem cell injections are popular amongst many Hollywood celebrities since they are easily and quickly done, do not result in bruising or swelling, and early results are visible within a few days, which makes it an ideal makeover treatment prior to events such as the Academy Awards. The secrets of stem cell facial injections are conquering the world.

17

The Recommendations

As a patient and potential consumer interested in stem cell therapies, it is very difficult to find the forest because of all the trees (a German saying). The internet is full of advertisements for stem cell therapy; the news is filled with astonishing study data and unexpected individual results accompanied by repeated warning statements from the FDA and others against using nonapproved therapies, which some people are willing to pay a lot of money for.

How do you work through all the advertisements, the basic research results, and the naysayers in doctors' offices to understand the real scenario in which someone might be a candidate for stem cell therapy without increasing your risks?

For potential patients, I suggest the following:

1. Get informed. One example is to read this book, which gives you more information than anyone has provided so far on the topic of stem cell therapy as an inside scoop on research, clinical studies, patient and physician interests, and regulatory requirements.

2. Do not believe in anything advertised on stem cell companies' websites.

3. If you talk to a stem cell company, ask about the physician(s) involved with the company. In particular, look up their physician license status on the state medical boards' websites, which will also show you if any state-board-initiated investigations are ongoing or were filed in the past.

4. Check the physician's qualifications. Are they board-certified in their field of expertise? I never would rely on any consumer reviews, which are often made up and really have no professional quality meaning, whatsoever. Does the physician work in or with a group that has a good reputation? Is the physician privileged at high-level medical institutions/hospitals (who usually do an intensive background check before they let someone in)?

5. Check out the physician's academic reputation. Do they have published scientific papers in their field? Are they participating in high-level research studies? This can easily be checked by going on PubMed.gov and typing the physician's last name followed by first-name initials in the search box. Every single publication they have coauthored in a reputable medical or scientific journal will appear.

6. Ask about the origin/source of the stem cells. Which lab produced them? What kind of cells are they? How are they administered? How many cells are used? What are the regulatory processes the lab goes through before the cells go to the patient? How do they ensure that the cells or cell products are viable?

7. How many patients have been treated in a similar way with the same product by this group/physician before? Where is the outcome data, and is anything published? What are the short-term and long-term side effects—if any?

8. Does the company have an IRB-approved study in place for the procedure?
9. Did the company apply for or receive an investigational new drug application?
10. What are the detailed costs, including physician fees, cell materials, technician costs, etc.?

In addition, there are certain red flags that tell you to avoid treatment from a group or physician:

1. If someone tells you that the stem cell therapy will cure your disease, run!
2. If someone tells you that there are absolutely no side effects, run!
3. If someone tells you that the therapy is FDA-approved (unless it is in the future), run!
4. If someone tells you that they have treated thousands of patients, but no published outcome data is available, run!
5. If someone gives you no information on their cell source, run!

Especially during the current COVID-19 pandemic, we have repeatedly learned that it is much better to trust scientists rather than believe the social media groups with secondary, nonscientific intentions.

Therefore, I suggest being careful and doing your homework before you agree to any nonstandard therapies. On the other hand, be curious, look into alternatives, be active, and believe me when I say that stem cell therapy represents a major medical breakthrough and will enormously change the face of medicine and age management in the near future.

18.

Stem Cell Secrets Revealed

In the previous chapters, I tried to create awareness about the pitfalls, false claims, and marketing tricks that often lack any scientific background. My intention behind this is for you to be aware of the facts and the myths of stem cell therapy. But there is strong evidence that stem cells have an enormous potential to help with the management of certain conditions and diseases with an almost unlimited indication for many acute and chronic illnesses.

Based on my own experience starting with basic research using stem cells and animal models to participation in multicenter trials as well as ongoing clinical studies, I present a list of conditions or diseases in this chapter for which our group has shown a significant improvement of the patient's conditions in many cases. Some of these have been scientifically analyzed and either have been published (such as our recent study for stem cell therapy for male erectile dysfunction) or submitted for publication in peer-reviewed, scientific journals. In other cases, we just have anecdotal successes, and our group is currently preparing the analysis of case studies and case series for publications.

The list below is in no way complete but represents our top ten picks for stem cell therapy use. It also does not mean that a single stem cell injection has cured any of these diseases. Based on my personal experience, I chose the conditions we have treated most over the last fifteen years with stem cells, and I present my personal rating of stem cell success. In this context, five stars means that every single patient my group has treated showed some success, four stars means that most patients treated showed some degree of improvement, three stars means that more than half of the patients treated had improvement of symptoms, and two stars means results were somewhat disappointing.

CONDITION	ROLE OF STEM CELLS	RATING
1. Heart Failure	A condition where the heart is weak. In particular, in advanced stages of reduced cardiac contractility, we have seen significant symptomatic improvement after stem cell therapy in addition to standard therapy for the management of heart failure.	****
2. Coronary Artery Disease (CAD)	In particular, in patients with multivessel coronary artery disease, meaning blockages in all arteries that are not amendable by stents or bypass surgery or even after the implantation of stents or bypass surgery and there is still the presence of diffused blockages with chest pains, stem cell injections showed significant improvement of symptoms even though the underlying condition cannot be cured.	****

3. Peripheral Vascular Disease	In particular, in patients with advanced peripheral vascular disease often as a result of long-standing diabetes in part in patients with nonhealing ulcers, stem cell injections have improved symptoms, helped heal open wounds and ulcers, and in several cases, helped to avoid foot or even leg amputations.	*****
4. Erectile Dysfunction	This is one of the indications for which we have used stem cell therapy the most due to the demand from patients. A systematic analysis of our data showed improvement of erectile dysfunction in every single individual to some degree (which does not mean cure but functional improvement).	*****
5. Facial rejuvenation	This represents one of the secrets in Hollywood that many celebrities have been using. The injection of stem cells using microneedle techniques all over the face stimulates skin rejuvenation and often makes the faces appear fresher and more viable and juvenile. For that reason, some individuals schedule this recurrently prior to auditions or award show appearances.	*****

6. Neurodegenerative diseases (strokes, Parkinson's disease, Lou Gehrig's disease, Alzheimer's disease, multiple sclerosis)	This represents a wide variety of different degenerative diseases of the brain and nerve tissue throughout the body often with significant weakness, paralysis, and a progressive decline of motor and sensory function finally leading to death. Several patients demonstrated a significant improvement of their motor neuron activities as well as a possible delay in the progression of the underlying disease.	****
7. Degenerative joint diseases (arthritis of the knees, the hips, or the shoulders)	Direct injections into the joints often relieves pain relatively quickly with astonishing symptomatic improvement lasting for several months after injections even in conditions with bone-on-bone situations where we did not expect anything.	*****
8. Chronic back pain	Chronic, especially low back, pain is usually caused by an inflammatory response of the surrounding tissues secondary to degenerative changes in the spine with compression of the nerves, for example, by bulging discs even though the underlying cause is not affected by any injection itself, most patients have a significant improvement of pain likely secondary to the anti-inflammatory effects of stem cells.	****
9. Chronic lung conditions (COPD, emphysema, asthma)	These conditions are irreversible and there is no curative therapy available. While some patients showed some improvement in functional capacity with less shortness of breath, others did not.	***

10. Hair loss	This is another area with significant improvements in most patients that might have to be repeated annually.	****

Besides these top ten picks for stem cell therapy, there are, of course, several other conditions for which stem cell therapy has shown significant improvements, in particular the adjunctive therapy of diabetes and many other conditions.

Interestingly, our group has seen amazing results in the treatment of **female sexual dysfunction**, which includes a conglomeration of different conditions, in particular one which is called female sexual arousal disorder. G-point injection of stem cells has shown promising results attributable to improved oxygen supply to the vagina and clitoris with subsequent increased function. Many of the patients we treated return for subsequent therapies, some of them on a yearly basis.

Infertility treatment has shown some possible benefits from stem cell injections according to a recently published study from China, where researchers injected stem cells directly into the female reproductive tract. Since this area is not within my frame of expertise, I personally do not have any clinical data to support this, but stem cell therapy might have a role in the adjunctive treatment of infertility in the very near future.

As mentioned earlier, stem cell transplantation as a therapy for certain forms of **cancer** is FDA-approved and has been widely established for approximately twenty years. Independent of that, many forms of cancer remain incurable and often lead to death. Current treatments include surgical removal of tumors, radiation therapy, chemotherapy that kills tumor cells with significant side effects on the entire organism due to cellular damage to healthy organs, and immunotherapy which is on the rise for certain subtypes of cancer. There are several preclinical and clinical trials underway to investigate the effectiveness of stem cell therapies, while others have warned against using stem cells in patients with underlying cancer due to concern for cancer-cell-promoting effects. I am personally reluctant to recommend any stem cell therapy in the presence of a current or recent cancer until further scientific data is available.

There are several other conditions from autism to recurrent muscle pain to **liver and kidney diseases** to **connective tissue diseases** and **immunologic disease** (such as lupus among many others), as well as acute **traumatic injuries** of tissue, muscles, joints, skin, and bones where we had good success rates.

The use of stem cells for **anti-aging** purposes, even though used by many, is very difficult to quantify since objective parameters are missing. In our practice, we often use measures for functional capacity, brain function, such as memory and concentration tests, as well as assessment of quality of life using established questionnaires, which in most patients all show significant improvement after a single stem cell injection. It goes without saying that these anecdotal reports need to be verified in controlled scientific studies.

In summary, stem cells are mostly effective in the adjunctive treatment of **vascular conditions,** whether it is **coronary artery disease, heart failure, peripheral vascular disease, or erectile dysfunction**, and the effects are mainly attributed to the fact that they are able to build new blood vessels and improve oxygenation of tissues at risk (**angiogenesis**).

The second large group of conditions in which stem cells show incredible benefits are those associated with **pain**, whether it is **chronic back pain, acute injuries,** or **degenerative joint diseases**, such as **arthritis** among others. The main effects on these conditions are attributable to the **anti-inflammatory properties** of stem cells, which often quickly relieve pain sensations and can last for a prolonged period of time.

The secret world of stem cell therapy, however, is unraveling.

Take-Home Message

- Physicians currently perform reactive medicine, which means diagnostic testing and therapy is aimed at improving symptoms that occur secondary to damage or loss of function.
- Regenerative medicine, on the other hand, aims to repair damaged tissue and restore functionality by recruiting the body's self-healing properties.
- We do lose the regenerative power of stem cells in our body with increased age.
- Certain organs, such as the heart and the brain (in contrast to the skin and the liver), do not regenerate on their own after damage occurs.
- Stem cell therapy represents one of the most promising advances in modern medicine, with the ability to partially induce regeneration of acutely injured or chronically damaged tissues.
- Most clinical studies testing stem cell therapy for different conditions have shown beneficial results with very little adverse events.
- Stem cell therapy outside the frame of ongoing clinical trials is not FDA-approved and is considered experimental.

- Stem cell therapy (with the exception of stem cell transplantation for certain forms of blood cancer) has not been shown to cure any disease, so far.

- There is a lack of information and misunderstanding in the general public about stem cell therapy.

- Consumers and patients interested in stem cell therapy are advised to gather objective information as outlined in this book or provided by regulatory agencies such as the FDA or professional medical societies rather than relying on marketing materials provided by commercial companies selling their services.

- Stem cell therapy is heavily investigated throughout the world and might change the practice of medicine in the very near future.

- Altogether, many of the secrets of stem cell therapy are outlined in this book, including the fact that stem cell therapy is not FDA-approved and necessary warnings not to trust marketing claims for cures of any disease. But we also would reemphasis the enormous potential of stem cells as regenerative therapy in general, and stem cells in particular, to delay processes of aging and improve overall health by treating chronic degenerative disease as well as acute injuries.

For more personalized information and consultations, please contact us directly at: www.drvonschwarz.com and www.heartstem.org.

About the Author

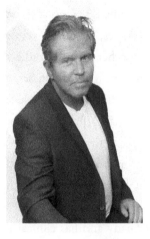

Dr. Ernst R. von Schwarz, MD, PhD is an Austrian-German-American physician and researcher who is a descendent of a Austrian-German family consisting of more than twenty doctors of medicine throughout the centuries. He grew up in Germany and received his Venia Legendi (Professor of Medicine) at the RWTH University of Technology in Aachen/Germany. He is a triple board-certified internist, cardiologist, and heart transplant cardiologist in Los Angeles. He is also a Professor of Medicine at Cedars Sinai Medical Center and a Clinical Professor at the David Geffen School of Medicine at UCLA and UC Riverside. Dr. Schwarz is a world-renowned clinical and academic heart specialist and serves as the Director of Cardiology and Director of the Heart Institute of the Southern California Hospital in Los Angeles, as well as Director and President of the Pacific Heart Medical Group in Murrieta, CEO of Dr. Schwarz Medical Institute of California, Medical Media Lab, and Medical Director of HeartStem, Inc.

Dr. Schwarz has published more than 150 scientific articles in international, peer-reviewed journals, several book chapters, and books in cardiology and medicine. He is a sought-after speaker at international scientific conferences worldwide. Dr. Schwarz is one of the thought leaders in modern future technologies, including stem cell therapies for chronic diseases for the heart and other organs. Students from universities from all over the world seek internships with Dr. Schwarz on an ongoing basis.

Dr. Schwarz studied medicine at the Universities of Vienna in Austria and the Philipps University in Marburg, Germany, and he worked and earned academic positions at the RWTH University of Technology in Aachen, Germany, the University of Ife in Ile-Ife in Nigeria, a Harvard affiliated hospital in Jeddah, Saudi Arabia, the University of Texas in Galveston, Texas, and Cedars Sinai Medical Center and UCLA. He resides in Los Angeles and Germany and has clinical practices in Los Angeles, Culver City, and Temecula, California.

Bibliography

This bibliography contains a list of selected publications mentioned in this book but does not represent the full list of manuscripts relevant to the context of this publication.

* indicates publications by the author of this book

1   *E. Skobel, A. Schuh, E.R. Schwarz, E.A. Liehn, A. Franke, S. Breuer, K. Günther, T. Reffelmann, P. Hanrath, & C. Weber, "Transplantation of fetal cardiomyocytes into infarcted rat hearts results in long-term functional improvement." Tissue engineering (2004): 10.
2   K.K. Hirschi, & M.A. Goodell, "Hematopoietic, vascular and cardiac fates of bone marrow-derived stem cells," Gene therapy (2002): 9.
3   Publication Committee for the VMAC Investigators (Vasodilatation in the Management of Acute CHF), "Intravenous nesiritide vs nitroglycerin for treatment of decompensated congestive heart failure: a randomized controlled trial," JAMA (2002): 287.
4   R.R. Arora, "Nesiritide: trials and tribulations. Journal of cardiovascular pharmacology and therapeutics" (2006): 11. J.D. Sackner-Bernstein, H.A. Skopicki, & K.D. Aaronson, KD, "Risk of

worsening renal function with nesiritide in patients with acutely decompensated heart failure," Circulation (2005): 111.

5 *E.R. Schwarz, S. Najam, R. Akel, N. Sulimanjee, S. Bionat, & S. Rosanio, "Intermittent outpatient nesiritide infusion reduces hospital admissions in patients with advanced heart failure," Journal of cardiovascular pharmacology and therapeutics (2007): 12.

6 T.J. Moore, H. Zhang, G. Anderson, & G. Alexander, "Estimated Costs of Pivotal Trials for Novel Therapeutic Agents Approved by the US Food and Drug Administration, 2015-2016," JAMA Intern Med. (2018): 178.

7 S.W. Junod, "FDA and Clinical Drug Trials: A Short History," US Food and Drug Administration (2008).

8 "What cells in the human body live the longest?" Science Focus.

9 M. Gadelkarim, A.I. Abushouk, E. Ghanem, A.M. Hamaad, A.M. Saad, & M.M. Abdel-Daim, MM, "Adipose-derived stem cells: Effectiveness and advances in delivery in diabetic wound healing," Biomedicine & pharmacotherapy (2018): 107.

10 K. Musunuru, F. Sheikh, R.M. Gupta, S.R. Houser, K.O. Maher, D.J. Milan, A. Terzic, J.C. Wu, & American Heart Association Council on Functional Genomics and Translational Biology; Council on Cardiovascular Disease in the Young; and Council on Cardiovascular and Stroke Nursing, "Induced Pluripotent Stem Cells for Cardiovascular Disease Modeling and Precision Medicine: A Scientific Statement From the American Heart Association," Circulation. Genomic and precision medicine (2018): 11.

11 L. Mazini, L. Rochette, B. Admou, S. Amal, & G. Malka, "Hopes and Limits of Adipose-Derived Stem Cells (ADSCs) and Mesenchymal Stem Cells (MSCs) in Wound Healing," International journal of molecular sciences (2020): 21.

12 S. Méndez-Ferrer, G.M. Ellison, D. Torella, & B. Nadal-Ginard, "Resident progenitors and bone marrow stem cells in myocardial

renewal and repair," Nature clinical practice. Cardiovascular medicine (2006): 3.

13 P. Menasché, V. Vanneaux, A. Hagège, A. Bel, B. Cholley, A. Parouchev, I. Cacciapuoti, R. Al-Daccak, N. Benhamouda, H. Blons, O. Agbulut, L. Tosca, J.H. Trouvin, J.R. Fabreguettes, V. Bellamy, D. Charron, E. Tartour, G. Tachdjian, M. Desnos, & J. Larghero, "Transplantation of Human Embryonic Stem Cell-Derived Cardiovascular Progenitors for Severe Ischemic Left Ventricular Dysfunction," Journal of the American College of Cardiology, (2018): 71.

14 D. Minteer, K.G. Marra, & J.P. Rubin, "Adipose-derived mesenchymal stem cells: biology and potential applications," Advances in biochemical engineering/biotechnology (2013): 129.

15 T.J. Povsic, C.M. O'Connor, T. Henry, A. Taussig, D.J. Kereiakes, F.D. Fortuin, A. Niederman, R. Schatz, R. Spencer, D. Owens, M. Banks, D. Joseph, R. Roberts, J.H. Alexander, & W. Sherman, "A double-blind, randomized, controlled, multicenter study to assess the safety and cardiovascular effects of skeletal myoblast implantation by catheter delivery in patients with chronic heart failure after myocardial infarction," American heart journal (2011): 162.

16 A. Malek, & N.A. Bersinger, "Human placental stem cells: biomedical potential and clinical relevance," Journal of stem cells (2011): 6.

17 J.H. Loughran, J.B. Elmore, M. Waqar, A.R. Chugh, & R. Bolli, "Cardiac stem cells in patients with ischemic cardiomyopathy: discovery, translation, and clinical investigation," Current atherosclerosis reports (2012): 14.

18 R.R. Makkar, D.J. Kereiakes, F. Aguirre, G. Kowalchuk, T. Chakravarty, K. Malliaras, G.S. Francis, T.J. Povsic, R. Schatz, J.H. Traverse, J.M. Pogoda, R.R. Smith, L. Marbán, D.D. Ascheim, M.R. Ostovaneh, J. Lima, A. DeMaria, E. Marbán, & T.D. Henry, "Intracoronary ALLogeneic heart STem cells to Achieve myocar-

dial Regeneration (ALLSTAR): a randomized, placebo-controlled, double-blinded trial," European heart journal (2020): 41.

19 R.R. Makkar, R.R. Smith, K. Cheng, K. Malliaras, L.E. Thomson, D. Berman, L.S. Czer, L. Marbán, A. Mendizabal, P.V. Johnston, S.D. Russell, K.H. Schuleri, A.C. Lardo, G. Gerstenblith, & E. Marbán, "Intracoronary cardiosphere-derived cells for heart regeneration after myocardial infarction (CADUCEUS): a prospective, randomised phase 1 trial," Lancet (London, England) (2012): 379.

20 *E. Skobel, A. Schuh, E.R. Schwarz, E.A. Liehn, A. Franke, S. Breuer, K. Günther, T. Reffelmann, P. Hanrath, & C. Weber, "Transplantation of fetal cardiomyocytes into infarcted rat hearts results in long-term functional improvement," Tissue engineering (2004): 10.

21 *E.R. Schwarz, F.A. Schoendube, S. Kostin, N. Schmiedtke, G. Schulz, U. Buell, B.J. Messmer, J. Morrison, P. Hanrath, & J. vom Dahl, "Prolonged myocardial hibernation exacerbates cardiomyocyte degeneration and impairs recovery of function after revascularization," Journal of the American College of Cardiology (1998): 31.

22 *E.R. Schwarz, J. Schaper, J. vom Dahl, C. Altehoefer, B. Grohmann, F. Schoendube, F.H. Sheehan, R. Uebis, U. Buell, B.J. Messmer, W. Schaper, & P. Hanrath, "Myocyte degeneration and cell death in hibernating human myocardium," Journal of the American College of Cardiology (1996): 27.

23 D. Buettner, "The Secrets of Long Life," National Geographic (2005).

24 T.A. Dong, P.B. Sandesara, D.S. Dhindsa, A. Mehta, L.C. Arneson, A.L. Dollar, P.R. Taub, & L.S. Sperling, "Intermittent Fasting: A Heart Healthy Dietary Pattern?" The American journal of medicine (2020): 133.

25 M. Barton, J. Grüntzig, M. Husmann, & J. Rösch, "Balloon Angioplasty - The Legacy of Andreas Grüntzig, M.D. (1939-1985)," Frontiers in cardiovascular medicine (2014): 1.

26 S. Roura, J.R. Bagó, C. Soler-Botija, J.M. Pujal, C. Gálvez-Montón, C. Prat-Vidal, A. Llucià-Valldeperas, J. Blanco, & A. Bayes-Genis, "Human umbilical cord blood-derived mesenchymal stem cells promote vascular growth in vivo," PloS one (2012): 7.

27 N. Nishiyama, S. Miyoshi, N. Hida, T. Uyama, K. Okamoto, Y. Ikegami, K. Miyado, K. Segawa, M. Terai, M. Sakamoto, S. Ogawa, & A. Umezawa, "The significant cardiomyogenic potential of human umbilical cord blood-derived mesenchymal stem cells in vitro," Stem cells (Dayton, Ohio) (2007): 25.

28 X. Li, Y.D. Hu, Y. Guo, Y. Chen, D.X. Guo, H.L. Zhou, F.L. Zhang, & Q.N. Zhao, "Safety and efficacy of intracoronary human umbilical cord-derived mesenchymal stem cell treatment for very old patients with coronary chronic total occlusion," Current pharmaceutical design (2015): 21.

29 L.R. Gao, Y. Chen, N.K. Zhang, X.L. Yang, H.L. Liu, Z.G. Wang, X.Y. Yan, Y. Wang, Z.M. Zhu, T.C. Li, L.H. Wang, H.Y. Chen, Y.D. Chen, C.L. Huang, P. Qu, C. Yao, B. Wang, G.H. Chen, Z.M. Wang, Z.Y. Xu, ... X. Hu, "Intracoronary infusion of Wharton's jelly-derived mesenchymal stem cells in acute myocardial infarction: double-blind, randomized controlled trial," BMC medicine (2015): 13.

30 P. Musialek, A. Mazurek, D. Jarocha, L. Tekieli, W. Szot, M. Kostkiewicz, R.P. Banys, M. Urbanczyk, A. Kadzielski, M. Trystula, J. Kijowski, K. Zmudka, P. Podolec, & M. Majka, "Myocardial regeneration strategy using Wharton's jelly mesenchymal stem cells as an off-the-shelf 'unlimited' therapeutic agent: results from the Acute Myocardial Infarction First-in-Man Study," Advances in interventional cardiology (2015): 11.

31 X. Li, Y.D. Hu, Y. Guo, Y. Chen, D.X. Guo, H.L. Zhou, F.L. Zhang, & Q.N. Zhao, "Safety and efficacy of intracoronary human umbilical cord-derived mesenchymal stem cell treatment for very

old patients with coronary chronic total occlusion," Current pharmaceutical design (2015): 21.

32 *M. He, & E.R. von Schwarz, E R, "Stem-cell therapy for erectile dysfunction: a review of clinical outcomes," International journal of impotence research (2020).

33 S.W. Kim, G.Q. Zhu, & W.J. Bae, "Mesenchymal Stem Cells Treatment for Erectile Dysfunction in Diabetic Rats," Sexual medicine reviews (2020): 8.

34 D. Bochinski, G.T. Lin, L. Nunes, R. Carrion, N. Rahman, C.S. Lin, & T.F. Lue, "The effect of neural embryonic stem cell therapy in a rat model of cavernosal nerve injury," BJU international (2004): 94.

35 Q.L. Hou, M.Y. Ge, C.D. Zhang, D.D. Tian, L.K. Wang, H.Z. Tian, W.H. Wang, & W.D. Zhang, "Adipose tissue-derived stem cell therapy for erectile dysfunction in rats: a systematic review and meta-analysis," International urology and nephrology (2017): 49.

36 J.Y. Bahk, J.H. Jung, H. Han, S.K. Min, & Y.S. Lee, "Treatment of diabetic impotence with umbilical cord blood stem cell intracavernosal transplant: preliminary report of 7 cases," Experimental and clinical transplantation: official journal of the Middle East Society for Organ Transplantation (2010): 8.

37 J.A. Levy, M. Marchand, L. Iorio, W. Cassini, & M.P. Zahalsky, "Determining the Feasibility of Managing Erectile Dysfunction in Humans With Placental-Derived Stem Cells," The Journal of the American Osteopathic Association (2016): 116.

38 R. Yiou, L. Hamidou, B. Birebent, D. Bitari, P. Lecorvoisier, I. Contremoulins, M. Khodari, A.M. Rodriguez, D. Augustin, F. Roudot-Thoraval, A. de la Taille, & H. Rouard, "Safety of Intracavernous Bone Marrow-Mononuclear Cells for Postradical Prostatectomy Erectile Dysfunction: An Open Dose-Escalation Pilot Study," European urology (2016): 69.

39 M.K. Haahr, C. Harken Jensen, N.M. Toyserkani, D.C. Andersen, P. Damkier, J.A. Sørensen, S.P. Sheikh, & L. Lund, "A 12-Month Follow-up After a Single Intracavernous Injection of Autologous Adipose-Derived Regenerative Cells in Patients with Erectile Dysfunction Following Radical Prostatectomy: An Open-Label Phase I Clinical Trial," Urology (2018): 121.

40 S. Al Demour, H. Jafar, S. Adwan, A. AlSharif, H. Alhawari, A. Alrabadi, A. Zayed, A. Jaradat, & A. Awidi "Safety and Potential Therapeutic Effect of Two Intracavernous Autologous Bone Marrow Derived Mesenchymal Stem Cells injections in Diabetic Patients with Erectile Dysfunction: An Open Label Phase I Clinical Trial," Urologia internationalis (2018): 101.

41 V. Protogerou, E. Michalopoulos, P. Mallis, I. Gontika, Z. Dimou, C. Liakouras, C. Stavropoulos-Giokas, N. Kostakopoulos, M. Chrisofos, & C. Deliveliotis, "Administration of Adipose Derived Mesenchymal Stem Cells and Platelet Lysate in Erectile Dysfunction: A Single Center Pilot Study," Bioengineering (Basel, Switzerland) (2019): 6.

42 *E.R. Schwarz, N. Busse, K. Mulholland Angelus, O. Ahmed, A.A. Schwarz, & P. Bogaardt, "Intracavernous Injection of Stem Cell-Derived Bioactive Molecules Improves Erectile Dysfunction," Journal of Men's Health (2021).

43 *A. Roberts & E.R. Schwarz, "An Analysis of Current Treatment Studies for COVID-19: Hydroxychloroquine, Remdesivir, and Convalescent Plasma," Submitted for publication under review (2021).

44 S. Singh, T. Chakravarty, P. Chen, A. Akhmerov, J. Falk, O. Friedman, T. Zaman, J.E. Ebinger, M. Gheorghiu, L. Marbán, E. Marbán, & R.R. Makkar, "Allogeneic cardiosphere-derived cells (CAP-1002) in critically ill COVID-19 patients: compassionate-use case series," Basic research in cardiology (2020): 115.

45 G. Lanzoni, E. Linetsky, D. Correa, S. Messinger Cayetano, R.A. Alvarez, D. Kouroupis, A. Alvarez Gil, R. Poggioli, P. Ruiz, A.C. Marttos, K. Hirani, C.A. Bell, H. Kusack, L. Rafkin, D. Baidal, A. Pastewski, K. Gawri, C. Leñero, A. Mantero, S.W. Metalonis, … C. Ricordi, "Umbilical cord mesenchymal stem cells for COVID-19 acute respiratory distress syndrome: A double-blind, phase 1/2a, randomized controlled trial," Stem cells translational medicine (2021).

46 *E.R. Schwarz, N. Busse, K. Mulholland Angelus, A. De La Torre, Y.J. Yu-Chi, S. Sung, B. Katlu, A. Shokoor, A.A. Schwarz, & P. Bogaardt, "Promising Benefit of Single Mesenchymal Stem Cell Injection in Critically ill Patients Suffering from COVID-19 Results from a Pilot Phase Randomized Controlled Study," Under review (2021).

47 P.A. Alvarez, E.R. Schwarz, R. Ramineni, P. Myatt, C. Barbin, C. Boissonnet, A. Phan, A. Maggioni, & A. Barbagelata, "Periprocedural adverse events in cell therapy trials in myocardial infarction and cardiomyopathy: a systematic review," Clinical research in cardiology: official journal of the German Cardiac Society (2013): 102.

48 *K.A. Thompson, R.P. Morrissey, A. Phan, & E.R. Schwarz, "Does the United States economy affect heart failure readmissions? A single metropolitan center analysis," Clinical cardiology (2012): 35.

A free ebook edition is available with the purchase of this book.

To claim your free ebook edition:

1. Visit MorganJamesBOGO.com
2. Sign your name CLEARLY in the space
3. Complete the form and submit a photo of the entire copyright page
4. You or your friend can download the ebook to your preferred device

Morgan James BOGO™

A **FREE** ebook edition is available for you or a friend with the purchase of this print book.

CLEARLY SIGN YOUR NAME ABOVE

Instructions to claim your free ebook edition:
1. Visit MorganJamesBOGO.com
2. Sign your name CLEARLY in the space above
3. Complete the form and submit a photo of this entire page
4. You or your friend can download the ebook to your preferred device

Print & Digital Together Forever.

Snap a photo

Free ebook

Read anywhere

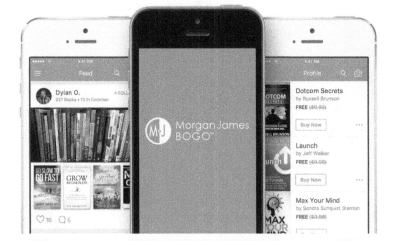

Printed in the USA
CPSIA information can be obtained
at www.ICGtesting.com
JSHW020041270224
58096JS00004B/232

9 781631 957079